Psychotropic Drugs:

a **M**anual for **E**mergency **M**anagement of **O**verdosage

by
Nathan S. Kline, M.D., F.A.C.P.
Stewart F. Alexander, M.D., F.A.C.P.
Amparo Chamberlain, R.N.

Medical Economics Company
Oradell, New Jersey 07649

Publisher's Notes

About the authors:

Nathan S. Kline, M.D., was a pioneer in the use of psychotropic drugs to treat mental illness. He is Director, Research Center, Rockland State Hospital, Orangeburg, N.Y.; Clinical Professor of Psychiatry at Columbia University; Director of Psychiatric Services, Bergen Pines County Hospital, Paramus, N.J.; and is engaged in the private practice of psychiatry in New York City.

Dr. Kline twice has been presented the Albert Lasker Award. He is noted as a clinician, educator, and researcher, having served in many advisory positions with major health organizations in the U.S. and abroad. He is on the Expert Advisory Panel of the World Health Organization, is adviser to the Committee on Mental Illness of the National Health Education Committee, and has served on numerous committees and advisory panels for the National Institute for Mental Health. Dr. Kline is President of the International Committee Against Mental Illness and a Foundations Fellow of the Royal College of Psychiatry.

Stewart F. Alexander, M.D., served as medical editor of the recently issued, "Hazards of Medication." He is director of medicine, Bergen Pines County Hospital; instructor in medicine at Columbia University College of Physicians and Surgeons; attending physician in medicine at Hackensack Hospital and Pascack Valley Hospital in New Jersey; and past president of the Academy of Medicine of New Jersey.

Amparo Chamberlain, R.N., is a clinical researcher and longtime associate of Dr. Kline at Rockland State Hospital.

Acknowledgments

The authors gratefully acknowledge the advice and assistance of Matthew Feldman, M.D., who served as pediatric consultant for this book.

Dr. Kline, particularly, acknowledges the advice and counsel of Dr. Bo Holmstedt, professor of toxicology, Karolinska Institute, Stockholm, Sweden; of the late Daniel H. Efron, M.D., Ph.D., National Institute of Mental Health; and of Prof. S. Moeschlin, Chief Physician, Buergerspital der Stadt Solothurn, Switzerland.

Mrs. Chamberlain acknowledges with appreciation the assistance of the Pharmacy Department of Rockland State Hospital.

Dr. Alexander expresses his appreciation for the assistance of Mrs. Effie A. Larsen, and Dr. Kline and Mrs. Chamberlain for the assistance of Mrs. Gloria Kistner and Mrs. Miriam Salzman in preparing the manuscript of this book.

The publisher and editors are indebted to Fred Witzig, Tenafly, N.J., for the patience and skill with which he designed the typography and format of this book.

About Sources

All the information about pharmaceutical products, their National Drug Code numbers, packaging, and manufacturers was accurate according to all sources and references available at the end of 1973.

How to Use This Book

This manual is intended to help you deal—step-by-step—with a victim of drug overdosage from the moment he is encountered until his physical condition is stabilized.

The information and instructions have been carefully selected, written, and typographically presented to make the manual easy, efficient, and effective to use.

It puts first things first.

You can start remedial measures immediately by starting at the front and proceeding directly through the book, following the advice applicable to the particular situation.

But don't wait for an actual emergency to find out how the manual works.

The more familiar you become with it beforehand, the more valuable it will be to you and the patient in an emergency situation.

Begin by consulting the detailed Table of Contents, printed both on page 6 and on the back cover. For laymen, the instructions on the next page are must reading.

Within each section of the manual, treatment details are arranged in order of importance. Degrees of importance within treatment sequences are indicated by varied sizes, weights, and color of type.

Specific individual pharmaceutical products have been cross-indexed to the major classifications of psychotropic drugs by means of identifying colors. Moreover, pages dealing with clinical signs and treatment for these major classifications of drugs are thumb-indexed.

Precise identification of the specific drug involved is rarely of vital importance during initial stages of treatment. But when a sample is available, the photo identification section will help you make an exact identification. In the first half of the section, drugs are pictured in alphabetical order according to brand name. The last half of the photo identification section divides drugs into major groups: capsules, white tablets, and colored tablets.

Specific details about dosages, packaging, uses, manufacturers, National Drug Code numbers, and street names for each drug are available from the section which consists of charts arranged in alphabetical order.

Finally, if you feel that you need additional advice, the last section of the book lists the telephone number and location of each Poison Control Center in your area.

Advice for Those Who Have Had No Medical Training

Although this book is intended as a guide for physicians, nurses, and first-aid or emergency squads, whoever first discovers a patient suffering from drug overdosage has a grave responsibility. The speed with which the situation is recognized may determine whether the patient lives or dies. No training is needed for these initial decisions.

What to do first in cases of drug overdosage depends chiefly on how well the patient is breathing.

If the patient is conscious and there is no problem with breathing

he or she should be taken as quickly as possible to the emergency room of the nearest hospital.

Few doctor's offices have all the equipment that may be needed for complete emergency treatment.

Do not waste time looking for a physician's office.

If there is any problem with breathing, call immediately for police assistance or an ambulance to move the patient to a hospital.

There should be at least ten reasonably deep breaths a minute.

Do not permit anything, internally or externally, to obstruct his breathing. If artificial respiration is needed and you know how to give it,

be sure the patient is on a hard surface like the floor—a bed is not a satisfactory place for artificial respiration.

Any drugs or bottles found near the patient should be taken with the patient to the hospital.

If no such material is found, look on the bedside table or in the medicine cabinet for a bottle or container carrying the name of the patient's physician or pharmacy. Fast accurate information about a person's medications and medical condition from either source could be lifesaving.

You Can Do What Is Boxed In Blue

If the patient is unconscious, call immediately for police assistance and an ambulance. Use an emergency number or enlist the telephone operator's aid to speed help. Again, make certain that nothing interferes with breathing. If you think the patient may vomit, the best position is face down on the floor with the head turned to one side. Hold the chin forward if breathing isn't easy.

Fear of social embarrassment must never influence your judgment. Concern for "what the neighbors might think" has needlessly cost many lives.

> **Never permit the patient, or his family, to talk you out of seeking immediate police and medical assistance.**

Let someone with expert knowledge decide whether or not the person belongs in a hospital.

When the ambulance arrives make certain that all drugs or bottles found and that other pertinent data, including the name of the patient's physician and pharmacy, if available, are taken to the hospital by the ambulance squad.

In this book the remedial measures a person without medical training may safely undertake in dealing with various situations are boxed in blue.

> **These are emergency measures only. They are not a substitute for prompt treatment in a hospital.**

However, the procedures outlined here can be crucial in keeping the patient alive if applied in a calm, vigorous, and sustained fashion.

**Protect the patient
Cover lightly
Turn on stomach if vomiting
Keep mouth and airway open and clean
Keep patient breathing
Do not use stimulants**

Table of Contents

Introduction

Nearly 250,000 known cases of drug overdosage occur annually. The 50,000 deaths that result are a toll greater than that for all infectious diseases combined.

Part of the reason for this toll undoubtedly is a lack of general knowledge about how to cope with such medical emergencies. This manual is intended to help remedy that situation.

Beyond dispute is the fact that many victims of drug overdosage are dependent solely on laymen for initial assistance. Therefore, information for nonmedical personnel has been included in this manual and, when appropriate, presented in nonmedical as well as "medical" language.

A warning: Whether you are inexperienced or have had some special training as a policeman, fireman or Red Cross trainee, the single most important rule is: **Recognize the limits of your competence. Do not get involved in using treatment methods beyond your skill.**

Physicians and registered nurses are well aware of the special limits to their competence. So this manual gives, for example, only the indications for dialysis, not details of technique, for only those with demonstrated skills and experience should attempt dialysis (removal of toxic substances directly from the blood).

Some of the recommendations in this basic manual may surprise those without expertise in dealing with drug overdosage. For example, the need to induce vomiting or to rouse the patient is of secondary importance and sometimes should be omitted completely in the interest of keeping the patient alive.

Observe these priorities in emergency management of cases involving drug overdosage:

— First, maintain respiration and adequate air exchange.

— Proper functioning of the cardiovascular system is of next importance.

— Treatment of convulsions, of abnormally high or low temperature, and other serious physiological problems are more important than relief of coma.

— Measures to increase the excretion, elimination, or breakdown of the toxic drug involved are important after support for vital functions has been taken care of.

The once popular use of cerebral stimulants has little place in management of drug overdosage cases today.

Finally, psychiatric considerations usually are important only after the preservation of life has been assured. Being last makes psychiatry far from least. Persons who have taken overdoses of psychotropic drugs deliberately are apt to do so again if not given psychiatric attention.

It's not sufficient just to preserve life; the reasons for overdosage must be determined. Some patients will explain that because of sleepiness or confusion more medication was taken than had been intended. Other

patients will admit having purposely taken excessive medication, but insist it was done to attract attention and
that actual suicide was not intended.

Either explanation may be true, but those involved,
especially the physician, should determine if there isn't
really some underlying disorder such as depression.
Moreover, there are other psychiatric disorders that can
lead to drug overdosage.

If a physician has any uncertainty about the emotional
factors in a case of drug overdosage, a psychiatric
consultation is necessary.

Accidental ingestion of drugs by children stresses a
vital and often broken rule: **All medication should be kept
out of reach of children.**

A few simple principles cannot be repeated too often:

— Physicians should prescribe only the quantity of
  medication a patient needs.

— Patients should be admonished to destroy all
  medication left after an illness.

— All medications should be dispensed in containers
  with safety caps.

— All medications should be labeled as to contents,
  dosage and instructions.

— Patients suspected of having suicidal tendencies
  should be supplied with only limited quantities
  of medication.

The format of this book is self-evident. Measures
concerned with preserving life are clearly labeled and are
listed in order of importance. Identification of the drug
involved is aided by picture grids, classifying each drug
by size, shape and approximate color.

In general the order of instructions is such that the
simple lifesaving procedures which anyone can do are
listed first and the more specialized medical procedures
listed last.

If the drug is known, the specific symptoms and
treatment recommendations are clearer, but treatment,
not drug identification, always takes priority.

If the drug is not known, or if a number of drugs have
been taken simultaneously, general treatment measures
should be followed.

We expect that there will be subsequent editions of
this manual as new drugs will inevitably produce new
problems. We would be most grateful if readers would
bring to our attention published or unpublished material
we might use to improve this emergency manual.

Respiratory Complications

Decreased respiration should be anticipated in all drug poisonings

Avoidance of respiratory tract complications is of greatest importance. Prevention is far better than later treatment. Minor problems or defects noted early and corrected promptly may prevent life-threatening situations later

Providing adequate oxygen is always the primary concern

Respiratory stimulant drugs, including caffeine (as in coffee), are of little value and should be avoided

Principles of Management

— Maintain adequate airway

— Remove excess secretions

— Maintain adequate ventilation of lungs

— Maintain acid-base equilibrium

— Protect lining of respiratory tract

— Protect against infection

Maintenance of Adequate Airway

1 Early recognition of respiratory difficulties is essential and can only be noted by constant observation and awareness of the hazard

2 Noisy air flow, snoring, crowing, gurgling, wheezing, supraclavicular or intercostal inspiratory retraction indicate obstruction and the need for immediate remedial action

— Tilt the patient's head backward

— Clean the mouth and throat with finger and/or suction

— Administer oxygen

— Pull lower jaw forward

— Use mouth-to-mouth resuscitation or hand-operated ventilator bag

— Insert oropharyngeal plastic tube of appropriate size

— Under direct laryngoscopy insert orotracheal cuffed tube. Inflated cuff must be deflated regularly at 2-hour intervals

Endotracheal intubation should be done only by personnel trained and experienced in this technique

— **Tracheotomy is not indicated unless all previous measures prove inadequate.** Laryngeal spasm may require puncture of the cricothyroid membrane or tracheotomy

— Administration of adequate amounts of oxygen early is essential, but is never a substitute for providing an adequate airway

3 Patients in coma or shock require constant checking to assure adequacy of the airway. Partial obstructions

may occur and contribute significantly to both coma
and shock

4   In prolonged coma or shock, the lack of normal
    activity often leads to obstructions of minor air
    passages to lung

— Change patient's position at least every hour or
  more often to prevent this
— Assist respiration if respiratory movement is
  inadequate
— Steam or vapor inhalation may be utilized
— Mucolytic agents may be added to air or oxygen
  systems

5   **Patients in coma or convulsion must be intubated
    with a cuffed endotracheal tube by experienced
    personnel prior to inducing vomiting or performing
    gastric lavage**

Removal of Excess Secretions

1   Clean patient's mouth with finger
2   Use gentle suction to clear oral space, oropharynx,
    nasopharynx, and laryngeal pharynx
3   Repeat suctioning as often as necessary. Keep
    suction tube clean

4   Do not use drugs to decrease salivation
5   Respiratory hygiene is essential
6   Mucolytic agents may be used, but are of only limited
    value

Maintenance of Alveolar Ventilation

1   Adequate oxygen exchange at alveolar level of the
    lung lining is essential. Inadequate oxygen supply
    produces respiratory acidosis, cardiac arrhythmia,
    and irreversible brain damage. Oxygen replacement
    must be immediate

2   Do not wait for onset of cyanosis to indicate that
    oxygen is not sufficient

3   Inspection and observation permit some judgment as
    to adequacy of ventilation exchange

4   Auscultation should help indicate adequacy of
    pulmonary ventilation

5   Arterial gas studies should be used freely if available.
    Patient's oxygenation is best monitored by this
    technique

6   Assisted respiration or controlled respiration equip-
    ment should be on hand before it is needed. Many
    satisfactory types of equipment are available. All
    persons expected to be able to provide emergency
    care should gain familiarity with the apparatus
    available

7   **Consultation with a skilled inhalation therapist should
    be sought if available**

8   The use of oxygen is not a substitute for providing
    adequate ventilatory exchange

Maintenance of Acid-Base Balance

1   Overzealous ventilation may produce a respiratory alkalosis

2   An intravenous infusion should be started on every patient in coma or shock, so that the capacity for rapid intravenous therapy is established. If no therapy is necessary, the IV should be maintained on a keep-open basis at a nominal flow rate. Normal saline, 5% dextrose in distilled water or normal saline, may be used initially

3   Respiratory acidosis may develop rapidly

4   Electrolyte and arterial gas studies should be undertaken immediately for all patients in coma or shock

5   Treatment for coexisting hypotension, shock, cardiac or renal complications will modify acid-base replacement factors

6   Cardiac arrhythmia may rapidly and gravely modify acid-base balance

7   Most acid-base problems can be avoided by maintaining adequate alveolar ventilation

8   Deviations from normal should be corrected promptly, **but not overzealously**

Protection of Lining of Respiratory Tract

The lining of the respiratory tract is fragile and so must be protected from trauma, drying, thermal changes and chemical exposure

1   Suction must be gentle

2   Placement of oropharyngeal tube must be gentle

3   Endotracheal intubation should be under direct laryngoscopy and gentle. Cuff should be gently inflated, and should be deflated regularly at 2-hour intervals. Failure to do so will damage the lining of the trachea and even produce local necrosis. Air or oxygen mixture used must be humidified, especially if ventilation is assisted or controlled

Protection Against Infection

1   All management of tracheotomy must be with aseptic technique

2   Endotracheal management calls for constant clean technique with frequent deflation of the cuff

3   Respiratory hygiene must be meticulous and observed at all times by all persons in contact with the patient

4   Early and repeated cultures should be obtained from the respiratory tract

5   Chest X-rays should be taken frequently

6   Antibiotic therapy should be initiated early and vigorously and related to the organism present

7   **Most pulmonary infections are hospital engendered.**

Circulatory Shock

Shock in drug overdosage is rare. It is caused largely by oxygen deficiency and vascular bed pooling

1   Shock is ominous and of the gravest prognosis
The sequence is: hypoxia → acidosis → diminished cardiac function → forward failure
Prevent or correct with proper ventilation

— Establish an adequate airway

— Assure adequate air exchange, either spontaneous or supported

— Intubate where possible with cuffed endotracheal tube

2   Blood pooling is the result of enlargement of vascular bed without increase in blood volume. Pooling may be a result of drug overdosage or of secondary factors

— Prevent or correct blood pooling with appropriate transfusion, plasma expanders, or infusion

— Basic physiological supports are important

— Drug excretion or metabolic breakdown is best enhanced by relief of shock and restoration of circulatory dynamics

3   Other causes for shock must be considered and eliminated, i.e., hemorrhage, brain injury, acute myocardial infarction, sepsis

Routine Procedures in Management of Shock

1   Place patient in shock position (lying flat on back, face upward, feet elevated)

2   Assure adequate airway. Use suction if needed. Insure adequate air exchange, spontaneous or artificial

3   Use oxygen

4   Maintain body temperature by using blankets, extra clothing, heat cradles. Do not use direct external heat. It could aggravate shock or cause burns

5   Apply pressure bandages to extremities to support blood pressure

6   Monitor blood pressure, temperature, pulse and respiration

7   Take electrocardiogram

8   Maintain hydration

Fluid by mouth is rarely adequate in this critical state. Never give fluid by mouth to a stuporous or semi-stuporous patient. Intravenous fluids are more effective. Normal saline is safest fluid to use until absence of diabetes, etc., has been established, but it will maintain blood pressure only briefly. Only slightly more effective is 5% dextrose in normal saline or distilled water. Give adequate amounts, but do not overload cardiovascular system. If in doubt, monitor central venous pressure in a hospital

9   Use plasma expanders such as low molecular
    Dextran, or serum albumin solutions. Blood
    transfusion is last choice unless there has been a
    complicating hemorrhage or anemia

10 Vasopressors may be used if necessary; see detailed
    descriptions in paragraphs on hypotension below

11 Actively seek and correct any complicating or
    contributing factors

Hypotension in Drug Overdosage is Common

1   Hypotension is best managed with intravenous fluids

    Vasopressors ordinarily should not be used as they
    cause decreased blood flow to those vital organs
    where it is most needed in cases of psychotropic
    drug overdosage

    So avoid vasopressors except briefly at start of
    severe hypotension after blood volume deficit has
    been corrected

2   Blood pressure must be monitored continually

3   Most psychotropic drugs potentiate vasopressors
    If indicated, Levophed, Neo-Synephrine, or Aramine
    may be used
    Prepare sterile intravenous solution of either

—   norepinephrine (Levophed) 4 ml of a 0.2% sol. in
    1000 ml of normal saline, 5% dextrose in normal
    saline, or in 5% dextrose in distilled water

or

—   phenylephrine (Neo-Synephrine) 10 mg in 500 ml
    of normal saline, 5% dextrose in normal saline, or
    in 5% dextrose in distilled water

or

—   metaraminol (Aramine) 50 mg in 50 ml of normal
    saline, 5% dextrose in normal saline, or 5%
    dextrose in distilled water
    Monitor blood pressure constantly. Regulate speed
    of infusion to bring blood pressure up to a 90 to
    110 mm/Hg level. A micro drip to regulate the rate
    of infusion is helpful.

    Avoid
    Epinephrine
    Picrotoxin
    Metrazol

    Avoid
    All stimulants
    All analeptics

Convulsions

Possible Causes

1. Cerebral anoxia (inadequate oxygen supply to brain) resulting from

— poor ventilation of lungs
— respiratory obstruction by mucus or vomitus
— laryngeal spasm

2. Direct action of drug on the central nervous system

3. Pre-existing disease triggered by the acute episode

4. Head injury (often unsuspected)

5. Associated unsuspected disease

Remedial Actions to be Taken Immediately

1. Assure free passage of air to and from lungs

2. Apply mouth gag and tongue clamp

3. Keep patient from injuring himself by thrashing or falling. Use padded restraint if required to prevent self-injury

4. Remove excessive secretions from mouth, throat and nose. Maintain careful oral hygiene

5. Give mouth-to-mouth or artificial respiration if necessary

6. Administer oxygen during convulsion

7. Do not induce vomiting or do gastric lavage while patient is convulsing

8. Attempt to control convulsions until diagnosis can be made and specific therapy started

9. Monitor fluid intake

10. Monitor fluid output. It should total 1 to 3 liters every 24 hours

11. Control body temperature (See section on Temperature Disturbances p. 16)

12. Start intravenous fluids with 5% dextrose in half-normal saline

Drug Control of Convulsions

1. Do not try to control convulsions with drugs until oropharyngeal secretions have been suctioned, adequate ventilation assured, oxygen administered, and respiration supported

2. Administer diazepam (Valium) 5 mg or 10 mg intravenously at a slow rate. (This is medication of first choice for children.) Take at least one minute to inject each 5 mg of drug. Do not mix with other drugs. Do not add to intravenous solution. If unable to administer safely intravenously, inject intramuscularly. (Most appropriate in tricyclic or MAOI overdosage)

3. Antispasmodic drugs often are effective in controlling convulsions

— Administer Akineton ½ ml (2.5 mg) intramuscularly
  or intravenously. Dosage may be repeated at
  one-half hour intervals, but do not give more than
  four doses in 24 hours **or**

— Artane 4 mg t.i.d. (only available p.o.) **or**

— Cogentin 1 mg per ml or 1 mg intramuscularly. No
  need for intravenous administration. Drug is
  cumulative. Increase by increments of 0.5 mg. Very
  useful in phenothiazine overdosage. Oral dose is
  1 to 4 mg b.i.d., starting with the smaller dose. In
  severe dystonia give intramuscularly

— Other antiParkinson drugs also may be used

4 Short-acting barbiturates may be administered unless
   the patient has been on a MAOI. Effective in tricyclic
   and phenothiazine overdosage, but use judiciously.
   May cause respiratory depression, particularly in
   children

5 Paraldehyde may be especially useful for children.
   Do not use paraldehyde if liver complications are
   present

6 Avoid succinylcholine (Anectine) unless given by
   anesthetist or physician experienced in its actions.
   This medication should be used when facilities and
   personnel needed for absolute control of respiration
   are fully available for duration of the medication's
   effects

Warning:

Diphenylhydantoin (Dilantin) and primidone (Mysoline)
have little or no place in the management of actual
convulsive seizure. Their use is to prevent subsequent
seizures

Death Can Occur From

Respiratory failure, especially during depression
following convulsion. (Support of respiration can help
prevent **anoxia** during prolonged spasm of
respiratory muscles)

Massive direct action of absorbed drug

Injudicious or overzealous therapy

Complications not directly associated with the drug
induced convulsion, such as a head injury, diabetes,
sepsis, etc.

Temperature Disturbances

Most psychotropic drugs can disturb the body's temperature regulating mechanism

Some drugs when taken alone or in combinations produce dangerous hyperpyrexia (dangerously high fever), which can cause permanent brain damage

Other drugs can cause a drop in body temperature to the near surrounding temperature which is usually lower than normal, thus resulting in hypothermia (abnormally low temperature)

In Hyperpyrexia (High Temperature)

1. Attempt fever reduction even while engaged in treating clinical signs of more emergent nature

2. Give cool drinks if compatible with ongoing drug overdosage treatment

3. Loosen or remove clothing to assure adequate ventilation of body

4. Apply wet towels

5. Sponge with cold water and vigorously massage skin to enhance spread of cooled cutaneous blood

6. Apply towels soaked in ice water and massage skin vigorously

7. Use ice-water tub bath followed by vigorous skin massage

8. Cool-water enemas may be useful

9. Use hypothermia machine, if available

10. Dialysis may be helpful in control of very severe hyperpyrexia

Fever increases
— cardiac load
— kidney load
— body requirements of oxygen
— body requirements of water
— body requirements of electrolytes
— metabolism by 10% for every 1° of fever

Elevated temperature has been an immediate cause of death in poisoning with tricyclics

In Hypothermia (Low Temperature)

1. Attempt to return temperature to normal even while engaged in treating clinical signs of more emergent nature

2. Give hot drinks where compatible with ongoing drug overdosage treatment

3. Apply blankets, bathrobes, sweaters, heat cradles (heated from outside)

4. Immerse body or extremities in water not over 42°C (107.6°F)

5. Do not apply direct external heat which could cause burns. Application of direct external heat also can produce circulatory collapse

6. Use hyperthermia machine, if available.

Coma

A patient in coma must be hospitalized so that intensive professional treatment can be started immediately
Maintenance of life and vital functions is the goal, not arousal of the patient
Do not use stimulants. More patients die of inappropriate therapy than from drug overdosage
Physiological support of vital functions (respiration, pulse rate and strength, blood pressure) until the drug can be metabolized or eliminated is the wisest therapy
Treatment varies with the degree of coma

Classification of coma

Grade I   **Light coma.** Patient responds to stimulation. There may be spontaneous or induced movements and groans
Vital signs are not altered. (If vital signs are abnormal, search for complications or coexisting damage or injury)

Grade II   **Deep coma.** However, reflex responses may be elicited. Vital signs are well maintained

Grade III   **Deep coma without response to any type of stimulus**
No reflex activities
Vital signs and functions usually are maintained initially; however, **prognosis is serious**

Grade IV   **Deep coma which persists for 24 hours or longer,** or coma in which vital functions become impaired. **Prognosis is serious**

Management of Coma

1   Assure adequate ventilation

— Observe respiratory pattern

— Keep patient on side, head extended, mouth to side with tongue forward

— Keep mouth, throat, and nasal passages free of mucus, vomitus, etc. Use suction if necessary

— Be prepared to give artificial respiration (e.g. when rate is below 10 respirations per minute)

— Insert a pharyngeal airway

— Be prepared to administer oxygen as indicated

— Intubate, where possible, with cuffed endotracheal tube. This should be done for first 48 hours of coma duration, **but only by trained personnel.**
(Cuffed endotracheal tube should be in place before lavaging patient in coma)

— **Check lung bases by auscultation to verify adequacy of ventilation**

2   **Treat shock if present**
3   Identify the drug taken, if possible

→

4 Rapidly, but diligently, search for other illness, disease or injury

5 Keep patient in horizontal position if he is not in shock. Turn every 30 minutes. Give skin care to avoid decubitus ulcers

6 Systematically observe and record
— Temperature, pulse, respiration, and blood pressure
— State of consciousness
— Skin color
— Fluid intake and output
— Corneal and patellar reflexes. These can indicate depth of coma
— Response to noxious stimuli (e.g. pain)

7 Pass indwelling catheter and monitor urine flow

8 Perform gastric lavage unless drugs were taken parenterally, or if oral ingestion was not recent

9 Secure stat blood chemistry, blood count and blood gases

10 Start intravenous infusion of 5% dextrose in ½ normal saline. Relate flow rate and amount to age, weight, state of dehydration, and other known disease or injury. (Average initial rate for adult is 20 drops a minute until adequate appraisal of patient can be made)

11 Maintain nutrition of patient intravenously, replacing fluids lost. If compatible with other treatment, tube feed when coma continues more than 48 hours and if kidney function is satisfactory

12 If muscle weakness and ECG changes point to a low blood potassium, give 10 Gm of potassium chloride in solution by gastric tube.
Do not give potassium chloride if there is renal failure without first checking the extent of potassium deficiency and renal output

13 Give procaine penicillin intramuscularly if there is a fever of prolonged coma, unless hypersensitivity is known or suspected. If in doubt, use a broad spectrum antibiotic

14 If use of a vasopressor is absolutely required, use one not contraindicated in overdosage of particular drug ingested. Give only enough to maintain near normal blood pressure and only as needed (First see section on Shock p. 12)

15 If coma persists, consider whether dialysis might be of benefit

Every case of coma should be classified and specific neurological and physiological phenomena should be monitored and recorded accurately

Reappearance of coma after patient seems to have improved may be the result of further absorption of drug remaining in intestines. When blood pressure rises from hypotonic levels and intestinal activity is resumed, further absorption will occur. **Also consider the possibility of subdural hematoma**

MAO Inhibitors: **Coma is light and of the type called "coma vigil." If coma is deep, suspect ingestion of a combination of drugs**

Doriden: Coma is apt to persist for days

Meprobamate: There is a rough estimate that adult patient will be in coma as many hours as he or she has taken tablets (400 mg) in excess of 20. Alcohol and drug combination overdosage is not infrequent

Skull fracture, epidural and subdural hemorrhage are critical injuries often overlooked in cases of coma caused by psychotropic overdosage

Pneumonia, sepsis, meningitis, and diabetes are the most commonly overlooked medical complications in cases of coma caused by psychotropic overdosage.

Drug Elimination: Gastric Mechanism

Emesis (vomiting) and lavage technique must be related to age and size of patient

Unless patient is comatose, convulsing or physiologically depressed, induce vomiting as rapidly as possible by

1   Irritating back of tongue or throat with spoon or finger

2   Giving glass of salt water (1 tablespoon/1 glass). Do not give more than 1 or 2 glasses and do not repeat. Irritate back of tongue after each glassful. If salt isn't available, use plain water

3   Giving 1 tablespoon **Syrup of Ipecac** (not fluid extract) followed by 1 or 2 glasses of water, milk or fruit juice

In Any Case

4   Give activated charcoal (50 Gm/500 ml water). Use enough charcoal to make a slurry the consistency of thick soup. Each gram of this adsorbs 100-1000 mgs. If Ipecac is used, give charcoal only after Ipecac has been tried, otherwise Ipecac will be adsorbed

5   Keep patient's head down during vomiting

6   Save vomitus for laboratory analysis

7   If other methods fail, consider subcutaneous Apomorphine (0.03 mg/lb body weight). The vomiting thus induced can be terminated by giving Lorfan intramuscularly (0.01 mg/lb body weight) one minute after onset of emesis

8   **Do not use Apomorphine in presence of physiological depression**

9   **Do not use central-acting emetics in phenothiazine overdosage.** Phenothiazines are strongly antiemetic

10   For children, vomiting is usually more efficient than lavage

Gastric Lavage

Before lavage, intubate comatose, unconscious or convulsing patients and those undergoing respiratory difficulties. Aspiration pneumonitis is a dangerous complication. To prevent it, use a cuffed endotracheal tube. If left in place, deflate every 2 hours for 15 minutes. Do not overinflate the tube as pressure can produce tracheal necrosis. Auscultate the abdomen. Absence of bowel sounds suggests continuation of lavage as absorption is very likely delayed

1   Aspirate gastric content before and after each wash. Save initial aspirate for laboratory analysis

2   Lavage where possible with normal saline using a wide-bore Ewald tube. Saline washes prevent water intoxication especially in children

3 Wash each time with small volumes (100 to 500 ml and never more than 2 glasses) lest stomach contents be pushed through pylorus. This is especially important with the first lavage

4 Use charcoal slurry in up to 400 ml of water for first wash where possible

5 Lavage until clear. Usually not more than 3 or 4 times

6 **Catharsis (Do not use cathartics unless reasonably certain no electrolyte imbalance exists. Measure electrolytes first if in doubt)**

   a. Before removing tube introduce a solution of sodium sulfate (30 Gm in 250 ml water—adult dose in absence of diarrhea) and leave in stomach as a cathartic. (Sodium sulfate is less toxic than magnesium sulfate especially if renal function is impaired although it may cause hypernatremia)

   b. In overdosage with lipid soluble drugs (e.g. barbiturates, amphetamines) lavage last with 50 ml aliquots of castor oil using a Toomey syringe for introduction and withdrawal. Remove with saline wash. Some castor oil will enter the intestine and act as cathartic

7 In poisoning with tricyclics (imipramine and related drugs), do not remove lavage tube. Repeated lavage at 1-hour intervals is advisable because of

— low plasma levels

— high rate of drug excretion in stomach

— drug's atropinic effect inhibits peristalsis so that lavage is useful long after drug is ingested

8 In poisonings with phenothiazines (Thorazine, etc.) lavage is especially useful. These drugs, though rapidly tissue bound, are water soluble. There is delayed gastric emptying so lavage has greater opportunity to remove unabsorbed portions

The "Scandinavian School" feels that absorption of a drug is increased by lavage and that poison is pushed into small intestine. They also report finding washing additives in lungs. Both of these complications may be minimized, however, with careful technique.

Drug Elimination: Renal Mechanism

The kidney is the most important organ in elimination of absorbed psychotropic drugs. Its function must be rapidly encouraged, protected, and enhanced. Drugs may be excreted unchanged or as metabolic products

Excretion depends on

— passive glomerular filtration
— active tubular secretion
— active tubular re-absorption
— passive tubular diffusion

Water Diuresis

Water diuresis increases excretion

Fluids are the best diuretic

Fluids by mouth are preferable if patient is conscious and not nauseated or vomiting

Never give fluids by mouth to a stuporous or semiconscious patient

Regurgitation or vomiting with aspiration can be lethal

Intravenous fluids are necessary in stupor, semi-coma, coma or agitation

1   Choose fluid in relation to all factors known, i.e., age, weight, state of hydration, other diseases present, fluid and electrolyte balance

2   Measure renal output with indwelling catheter and monitor per minute or multiple minute flow. Do not catheterize if patient is alert enough to permit accurate urine recovery

3   Avoid overload of cardiovascular system and try to avoid pulmonary edema

4   If in doubt, monitor central venous pressure in hospital

Osmotic Diuresis

1   Mannitol

— 100 ml 10% Mannitol slowly given intravenously

— Follow with 5% glucose in normal saline in 1000 ml units

— Add KCl to intravenous solution after diuresis. Amount determined by degree of diuresis, level of serum potassium, and/or height of T wave in electrocardiogram

— Maintain careful records. Mannitol, though it may be effective, is limited in its usefulness. It usually should not be continued for more than 2-3 days

2   Urea

— **Cannot be used in patients with renal insufficiency or renal failure;** has limited usefulness

— Give intravenously, hourly, for 4 hours: 300 ml Ringer's lactate with 80 ml 50% urea solution (in isotonic saline)

— When urine excretion reaches 500 ml/hr, continue with 600 ml Ringer's lactate and 10-30 ml 50% urea solution hourly. **Re-evaluate at 4-hour intervals**

— **If retention of more than 50-60 ml fluid per hour occurs, procedure must be discontinued**

— **Measure hourly intake and output and record**

— **Keep blood urea nitrogen under 200 mg per cent**

— Make serum calcium, sodium and potassium studies throughout treatment. Replace these as needed

Chemical Diuretics

Furosemide and ethacrynic acid are most potent

Patient must be well hydrated

May be used in conjunction with or following Mannitol

Fluid and electrolytes must be monitored

Potassium loss must be expected and judiciously replaced

Dosages
Furosemide (Lasix)—40 mg intramuscularly (or intravenously slowly). If no diuresis, may repeat in 2 hours as 80 mg intramuscularly (or intravenously slowly). Consultation suggested if higher doses are required
Ethacrynic Acid—50 mg reconstituted in 50 ml of 5% dextrose in water or 5% dextrose in normal saline; give intravenously over course of 10 minutes. Thiazides and Spironolactone may be given orally only; are slower, less effective
Mercurials are best avoided

Acid or Alkaline Therapy

— Are of more theoretical than practical use. In phenobarbital overdosage alkalinization may be useful as phenobarbital has a high pK and raising the pH increases its dissociation and excretion

— pH and blood gases must be monitored and deviations from normal corrected

— Acid forced diuresis is useful in amphetamine intoxication

Injudicious Diuretic Therapy

Without adequate fluid replacement diuresis is poor therapy. It produces dehydration, pulmonary complications and hypoxia

Failure to Effect Diuresis

Implies renal failure, and alternate methods of therapy must be considered including dialysis (see section on Dialysis p. 24)

Indwelling Catheter

(Foley or other) is mandatory to monitor urine output in the critically ill or comatose patient.

Drug Elimination: Dialysis

Dialysis is an extra-renal means of removing psychotropic drugs or other toxic products from the body. It may be a lifesaving procedure

There are two types

Hemodialysis
Peritoneal dialysis

Neither should be used until other appropriate measures have been initiated

When to use

1   In Grade III and Grade IV coma
2   In renal shutdown or impaired renal function
3   In life-threatening overdoses complicated by

— pulmonary edema
— heart failure
— circulatory collapse
— significant liver disease
— major metabolic disturbance
— uremia

4   Early in cases where there is certainty of very large overdosage that cannot otherwise be removed

Which to use

Hemodialysis	Peritoneal Dialysis
More potent	Rapid to institute
More reliable	Less reliable
May be used in Grade III and IV coma	May use in Grade II and Grade III coma
Requires special equipment	Simple to perform: no special equipment required
Requires trained personnel	
Requires sophisticated laboratory capability	Basic laboratory facilities must be available
Usually requires blood	Fluids are commercially distributed and more readily available
Greater cardiovascular complications	Infections are a hazard
More expensive	

How to use

1   **Physician must be thoroughly familiar with technique and its possible complications**
2   Techniques are easy to learn
3   Dialysis must be used in combination with

   a. Full range of sustained supportive measures, including

   adequate fluids

adequate survey

effective ventilation, spontaneous or supported

frequent and adequate suctioning

Foley catheter and urine monitoring

continuing observation with monitoring of vital signs and depth of coma

b. Diuresis enhancement, using

parenteral fluids

glucose and saline

Mannitol infusion

Solutions are commercially available. The principle is to use a dialysis solution similar to interstitial fluid

Some Common Psychotropic Drugs That Can Be Removed to Some Degree by Dialysis

acetophenetidin	
alcohol	
amphetamines	Benzedrine, Edrisal
aspirin	
barbiturates	Amytal, Sombulex, Noctopan, Nembutal, Seconal, Tuinal
bromides	Neurosine
chloral hydrate	Noctec, etc.
chlordiazepoxide	Librax, Librium
diphenylhydantoin	Dilantin, Mebroin
ethchlorvynol	Placidyl
glutethimide	Doriden
heroin	
isocarboxazid	Marplan
meprobamate	Miltown, Equanil, etc.
methamphetamine	Desoxyn, etc.
methaqualone	Quaalude, Somnafac
methyprylon	Noludar
paraldehyde	
pargyline	Eutonyl
tranylcypromine	Parnate
phenelzine	Nardil
reserpine	Serpasil

Effectiveness of Dialysis in Psychotropic Drug Overdosage

analgesics	rarely needed
antihistamines	rarely needed
hypnotics and sedatives	may be lifesaving
minor tranquilizers	generally useful
monoamine oxidase inhibitors	useful
phenothiazines	of little value; may be used
tricyclics	difficult; may not be useful

Dialysis is usually not recommended for phenothiazines and tricyclics

Hazards

They are multiple and should be evaluated prior to initiation of the procedure →

1 **Excessive potassium washout**
— Hypokalemia may be fatal
— Potassium levels must be monitored

2 **Fluid overload** can precipitate heart failure

3 **Infections** are a major danger

4 **Irreversible tissue changes** may preclude recovery

Trained personnel and facilities for dialysis are necessary in all centers where overdosages are expected to be treated

Dialysis may be lifesaving, but never is the first measure to be instituted. It requires skilled professional supervision and can only be used in conjunction with all other vital and indicated treatment measures

(New dialysis techniques including use of resins and adsorbatives are being developed, but are of investigative interest only at this time.)

Clinical Signs and Treatment

Drug Combinations

The problem of drug overdosage is frequently complicated by ingestion of more than one psychotropic drug at the same time or in close sequence. The combined use of drugs and alcohol unfortunately is also common and dangerous.

In combined drug overdosage the classical signs and symptoms of overdosage with one drug may be altered or masked by the effect of the other drug or drugs present. An otherwise safe dose may prove lethal in combination with another psychotropic drug or with alcohol. Unfortunately, this important fact is not well known. Coexisting disease, exposure, and serious visceral or cerebral injury may further obscure the clinical picture.

The bizarre and complicated symptoms resulting may confuse even a competent physician. However, the preservation of life and of vital functions is always more important than immediate specific drug identification.

Amphetamines and Related Drugs

(Drug could have been ingested, injected, inhaled, or applied to mucous membrane)

Clinical Signs

Tachycardia, chest pains
Restlessness, irritability
Dizziness
Nausea, vomiting
Metallic taste
Dilated pupils, blurred vision
Apprehensiveness, confusion
Abdominal cramps, flatulence, diarrhea
Headache
Urine retention
Pallor, flushing, cyanosis
Chills
Gasping respirations
Profuse sweating
High fever (in children may reach 109°)
Tremors
Hyperactive reflexes, spasms
Hallucinations, delirium, fear (particularly with inhalation or injection of deteriorated [pink] epinephrine)
Hypertension or hypotension. The blood pressure which may be high initially can go down to subnormal accompanied by absence of urinary output
Cardiac arrhythmias
Circulatory collapse
Convulsions
Coma
Respiratory failure
Note: Subcutaneous or perivascular injection of some of these drugs causes sloughing at site of injection

Treatment

1. Give artificial respiration or oxygen as needed

2. Give milk, tap water or activated charcoal (50 Gm in 500 ml of water) to delay absorption

3. Provoke vomiting in conscious patients. Guard against inhaling vomitus

4. Perform gastric lavage followed by saline cathartic (sodium sulfate) 30 Gm (about 1 ounce) in 250 ml of water (about 1 glass)

5. Control convulsions with cautious administration of open-drop ether

6. Sedate with chlorpromazine 0.5 to 4 mg/kg using smaller dose when drug has been ingested in combination with a barbiturate

7. Treat shock conventionally

8. Thirst is apt to be marked but do not give excessive fluid because of risk of pulmonary edema →

9   Monitor fluid and electrolyte balance
Catheterize when necessary

10   For systemic reactions administer Regitine
5 mg slowly IV or Phentolamine HCl 100 mg
orally or chlorpromazine 0.5-4 mg/kg

11   In severe cases of hypertension
extracorporeal dialysis has been
recommended by some clinicians

12   Use sponge baths, ice packs to control fever

13   Keep patient quiet in darkened surroundings

14   Protect patient from self-injury; use padded
restraint and bed.

Antianxiety Agents

Clinical Signs

Drowsiness
Lethargy
Nystagmus (rapid, involuntary movement of
    eyeball); diplopia (double vision)
Blurred vision, pinpoint pupils
Weakness, lassitude, muscle relaxation
Tinnitus (ringing or buzzing noise in ears)
Mental confusion, hallucinations
Diminished reflexes, poor coordination
Hyperactivity, convulsions in some cases
Paradoxical excitation, rage in others
Hypotension/shock
Coma with cyanosis
Respiratory depression

These drugs potentiate

Alcohol
Anesthetics
Other sedatives, hypnotics

And are potentiated by

Narcotics
Monoamine oxidase inhibitors
Tricyclics
Barbiturates
Phenothiazines

Treatment

1   Maintain open airway. Administer artificial
    respiration or oxygen when necessary

2   Retard drug absorption by giving tap water
    or milk, 100-500 ml usually 2 or 3 times.
    Or use activated charcoal (50 Gm in 500 ml
    water)

3   Induce vomiting in conscious patients

4   Start gastric lavage (use cuffed endotracheal
    tube in unconscious patients). Leave solution
    of sodium sulfate (30 Gm/250 ml) in stomach
    as cathartic

    Meprobamate and diazepam (Valium) are not
    water soluble, so best results are obtained if
    gastric elimination attempts are started soon
    after drug ingestion. Benzodiazepines
    (Valium, Librium) generally have long plasma
    half-life, so hemodialysis may prove necessary

5   Hypotension/coma: maintain fluid balance
    with intravenous fluids. **These patients are
    susceptible to congestive heart failure
    and pulmonary edema.** Keep this in mind
    when volumes of intravenous fluids are
    administered in attempts to control hypo-
    tension or for diuresis
    Caution: during coma and hypotensive state
    all meprobamates may not be absorbed
    from intestinal tract. With return of normal
    circulatory functions the residual drug is

absorbed, thus causing a reappearance of the poisoning syndrome

— Therefore
Keep an open vein
Do not relax treatment
Observe patient for at least 72 hours after drug ingestion

(A rough rule has been suggested regarding coma in meprobamate poisoning: adult patient will be as many hours in coma as he has taken tablets [400 mg] in excess of 20)

If coma does not respond to routine measures, one of the following procedures may be tried

— Osmotic diuresis
— Mannitol diuresis
— Peritoneal or hemodialysis

Supportive nursing care should include

> Cold sponges
> Ice packs for fever
> Positional changes
> Monitoring of vital signs
> Fluid intake and output control

Warnings:

Do not give epinephrine. Its action may be paradoxical

Do not administer barbiturates to patients exhibiting signs of stimulation.

Antihistamines

Clinical Signs

Dilated pupils (mydriasis)
Dry mouth
Flushed face
Drowsiness
Ataxia (unsteady gait), tremors
Hallucinations
Convulsions (intermittent tonic-clonic)
Fever
Stupor on to coma
Cardiorespiratory collapse

Treatment

1   Retard absorption by giving charcoal slurry
    (50 Gm/500 ml of water)
    (See Gastric Elimination p. 20)

2   Gastric lavage (100-500 ml). If possible use
    potassium permanganate solution 1:2000.
    Usually 2 or 3 times

—   Leave saline cathartic in stomach after lavage

3   Maintain blood pressure

4   **Control convulsions with cautious use of a
    short-acting depressant such as Valium, a
    barbiturate or ether**

5   Treat respiratory depression conventionally
    with artificial respiration and oxygen

6   Do not use stimulants

7   Do blood studies

8   If agranulocytosis develops, give a broad
    spectrum antibiotic

9   To maintain urine volume at 200-400 ml/hour,
    Mannitol diuresis may be needed
    (See Renal Elimination p. 22.)

AntiParkinson Drugs

(These agents also are used with or to alleviate
certain side effects of phenothiazine and
phenothiazine-like drugs)

Clinical Signs

Dilated pupils with loss of light reflex and
    accommodation
Increased intraocular tension
Blurring of vision; sensitivity to light
Dry mucous membranes
Difficulty in swallowing (because of dryness of
    mucous membranes)
Thirst
Rapid pulse, weak pulse; palpitation
Hot, dry skin (no sweating), flushing
Fever (may reach 109°F in children)
Confusion, disorientation, delirium, visual
    hallucinations
Speech disturbances
Talkativeness, excitability
Blood pressure initially elevated
Urine retention, difficulty in urinating
Abdominal distention
Rapid respirations becoming slow and shallow
Convulsions
In cases of severe intoxication, signs may
    progress to hypotension, paralysis and coma

Treatment

1   Give mouth wash to remove any drug
    remaining on mucous membranes

—   If drug was ingested give 250 ml milk or
    activated charcoal (50 Gm/500 ml water) or
    water if neither milk nor charcoal is available

—   Induce vomiting in conscious patients; guard
    against inhalation of vomitus

—   Perform gastric aspiration and lavage

—   Follow with saline cathartic (sodium sulfate
    30 Gm/250 ml water).
    Unconscious patients must be intubated
    before performing above procedures

—   Give fluids by mouth and intravenously
    (glucose)

—   Monitor electrolyte balance, fluid intake
    and output

2   Hyperactivity
    Manage with small doses of short-acting
    barbiturates, paraldehyde or chloral hydrate.
    Administer cautiously so as not to
    provoke respiratory depression

3   Convulsions
    Prevent biting or swallowing of tongue. Use
    mouth gag or padded tongue depressor

4   Fever
    Treat with cold sponges, ice packs or other
    methods to reduce temperature

5   Respiratory depression
    Manage with artificial respiration and oxygen

— Avoid central-acting stimulants

— Avoid morphine

6   Supportive measures

— Keep patient in quiet, darkened surroundings

— Catheterize where necessary

Special Dangers of AntiParkinson Drug Overdosage

Previous cardiac arrhythmia increases hazards

Spasm of sphincter muscles. Acute prostate
problems may be precipitated and cause
acute urinary retention.

AntiParkinson
Drugs

Barbiturates and Barbiturate-like Agents

Clinical Signs

Disorientation
Sleepiness, lethargy
Unsteadiness
Contraction of pupils of eyes; dilation may
    occur later
Dilation of pupil is characteristic of glutethimide
    (Doriden) poisoning
Deep coma (prolonged if there is cerebral edema)
Flaccid muscles
Absence of corneal and other reflexes
Increased or decreased temperature
Slow, shallow respirations
Anoxia, cyanosis
Fall in blood pressure
Shock
Moist rales in lower lung fields may be indicative
    of pulmonary edema in the comatose patient
**There always is a possibility of pneumonia
    associated with lung congestion of any
    duration**

Treatment

Treatment is concerned with avoiding respiratory,
pulmonary, and cardiovascular complications
as any one of these may cause death

1   Provide adequate airway

— Suction mucous secretions with rubber
   catheter; prevent aspiration

— Use oropharyngeal airway when necessary

— Place a cuffed laryngeal airway or do a
   tracheotomy when there is laryngeal stridor
   or edema. Be alert to and prepared for
   possibility of cardiac or respiratory arrest
   during intubation

— **Decompress cuff regularly at 2-hour intervals**

— Remove airway within 48 hours

2   Support adequate respiratory exchange

— Administer artificial respiration or oxygen
   (moistened) where needed

— Do not use stimulants. They can cause
   complications of a serious nature, e.g.,
   cardiac failure or arrhythmias, convulsions,
   renal injury or psychosis

— When absolutely necessary, use bemegride
   (Megemide) IV—50 mg doses at 3-5 minutes
   until improvement; ethamivan (Emivan) or
   methylphenidate (Ritalin), but only in quantities required to maintain minimal reflexes

3   Induce vomiting, but guard against aspiration
    of vomitus
—   In conscious patients give activated charcoal
    (50 Gm/500 ml water well shaken until all
    charcoal is wetted) by lavage tube if necessary.

—   Remove by emesis or lavage tube aspiration.
    Repeat procedure. (It has been reported that
    1 Gm of activated charcoal adsorbs 100 to
    1000 mg of toxic agents)

4   Gastric lavage (place cuffed endotracheal
    tube prior to lavage of unconscious patients)

—   Aspirate first and save contents for analysis

—   Use 100 ml to 500 ml amounts in lavage as
    specified above

—   Leave saline cathartic in stomach (30 Gm
    sodium sulfate in 250 ml water)

5   If drug has been injected, apply tourniquet
    and ice pack at site to slow absorption

6   Elimination essentially is renal with many of
    these drugs

—   Where renal function is not impaired,
    Mannitol diuresis may be instituted

—   Monitor and maintain electrolyte and fluid
    balance

—   Catheterize when indicated

    Detoxification is primarily by liver. Toxicity
    is accentuated by liver disease or liver
    impairment

Hemodialysis

When blood drug level is high in long-acting
barbiturate poisoning, hemodialysis has been
found useful

Both diuresis and dialysis are discouraged in
patients with

stubborn hypotension
pulmonary edema
impaired renal function

7   Hypotension, shock

—   Maintain blood pressure with intravenous
    fluids such as 5% glucose in saline, blood,
    or plasma

—   If there is no improvement in blood pressure
    after administering 1 liter of intravenous
    fluid, norepinephrine may be added to
    intravenous fluid, but add only enough to
    produce near normal blood pressure.
    Discontinue norepinephrine as soon as
    possible. Check reflexes regularly; they
    indicate severity of depression

8   **Pneumonia: Treat with appropriate
    chemotherapy**   →

9 Supportive Care

— Positional changes of patient at least every 2 hours are needed

— Elevate foot of bed to avoid aspiration of secretions

— Suction oropharyngeal secretions

— Use blankets in hypothermia. Do not use mechanical warming devices

— Use cold, wet towels to reduce elevated temperature

— Keep patient quiet, in darkened room where possible

— When indicated, manage hypnotic abuse withdrawal syndrome. (Phenobarbital may be useful.)

Monoamine Oxidase Inhibitors

Clinical Signs

Weakness, dizziness, **postural hypotension**
Excitability, hypertonia, spasticity eventuating in
    convulsions
Dry mouth
Nausea, vomiting
Mydriasis (dilated pupils), photophobia
    (abnormal sensitivity to light)
Stupor
Mental confusion and incoherence progressing
    to stupor, even coma
Neck stiffness
Ataxia, sluggish reflexes
Convulsions
Coma
Hypotension/shock
Hypertensive crisis as manifested by
    flushed face
    occipital headache radiating frontally
    neck stiffness
    nausea, vomiting
    photophobia
Hyperpyrexia
    Sweating with fever or with cold, clammy
    hands
Hypertension and fever are accompanied at times
    by twitching and myoclonic fibrillation of
    skeletal muscles, sometimes progressing to
    generalized rigidity and coma
Rapid heartbeat or slow heartbeat associated
    with dilated pupils and constricting chest pains
Very rapid breathing with congestion and
    occasional rhythm problems
Respiratory depression
Death may occur from
    respiratory failure
    circulatory failure
    intracranial bleeding
**Watch out for hypertensive crisis appearing
    concurrently with postural hypotension**
Clinical signs of overdosage may not appear for
    up to 12 hours after drug ingestion allowing
    for early treatment. Overdosage signs may
    continue 8-10 days after ingestion of drug.
    (The action of certain amines is markedly
    potentiated, since monoamine oxidase
    inhibitors block the enzymes which usually
    lead to amine catabolism. This is particularly
    so if amines are given parenterally)

Dangerous Combinations

1   With drugs that may precipitate a hypertensive
    crisis. (This may be fatal, the result of
    circulatory collapse or intracranial bleeding)

—   Parenteral use of sympathomimetic drugs,
    such as

    amphetamine
    epinephrine   →

norepinephrine

— **methyldopa or dopamine**

— **Large/parenteral doses of dibenzazepine derivatives,** such as desipramine (Pertofrane, Norpramine), amitriptyline (Elavil itself or found in Etrafon or Triavil)

— Large doses of certain proprietary drugs such as those used for cold, hay fever, or reducing which may contain a sympathomimetic agent

— Food high in tyramine, such as beer, wines (especially Chianti), fermented cheeses, pickled herring, chicken livers, yeast extract

— Food high in tryptophan, such as broad beans

2   With drugs possibly causing serious hypotension if used in high doses

— barbiturates
— narcotics
— analgesics
— alcohol
— thiazide diuretics
— phenothiazine compounds

Treatment

1   Maintain open airway.
Support respirations if necessary with oxygen or artificial respiration

2   Attempt removal of drug by vomiting,

gastric lavage, catharsis, and forced diuresis

3   Maintain hydration and electrolyte balance with intravenous fluids
Record intake and output

4   Therapy for Convulsions

— Correct shock or hypotension if present

— Barbiturates help relieve myoclonic reactions; **administer cautiously**

— Give intravenous phenothiazine for sedation

— Administer 10-15 mg succinylcholine chloride intravenously, very slowly and under strictly controlled ventilation

— Reduce fever with external cooling

5   Hypotension/shock/coma therapy

— Treat conventionally bearing in mind that MAOIs potentiate

— Watch rate of infusion; avoid sudden variations in blood pressure

— Plasma and plasma expanders are most valuable, since MAOIs block vascular bed response

— Vasopressors may be given very cautiously and only when all other measures have been used and found inadequate

— Binders and pressure bandages may be used to support blood pressure

6 Hypertension

— Use Phentolamine (Regitine) 5 mg intravenously
Or Pentolinium (Ansolysen) 3 mg subcutaneously
Administer slowly to prevent excessive hypotension
Do not give parenteral reserpine

— Continue treatment till homeostasis is restored; follow for at least 10 days; toxic effects may be prolonged

— Liver function tests should be performed initially and repeated in 4-6 weeks, if not sooner on indication

Special Notes

Use cautiously and only if necessary the following drugs

Barbiturates. Their use may result in apnea. A phenothiazine is better if sedation is needed

Vasopressors/stimulants. Remember tissues are already saturated with epinephrine

CNS depressants such as narcotics, Demerol, ethanol, anesthetics, atropine, papaverine, scopolamine, etc.

Cocaine or local anesthetics containing sympathomimetic vasoconstrictors.

Monoamine Oxidase Inhibitors

Narcotics

Clinical Signs

Pinpoint pupils (miosis) unresponsive to light
Nausea, vomiting
Dry mouth
Sweating
Hypothermia (lowered temperature), cold,
    clammy skin
Muscle twitching
Flaccid muscles
Marked respiratory depression
Slow, weak, regular pulse
Gastrointestinal and biliary tract spasms
Normal blood pressure except where there is
    oxygen deficiency
Convulsions in some cases (from codeine,
    Demerol, Apomorphine)
Unconsciousness, coma

Possible Complications

Pneumonia
Pulmonary edema

Treatment

1   Attend to respiratory emergency if present
    and maintain open airway

— **Give narcan (Naloxone) 0.4 mg intravenously,
intramuscularly, subcutaneously.** Repeat at
3-minute intervals. If no response is detected
after 3 doses, another drug is involved or
another disease or complication exists

— Administer Nalline 5-10 mg intravenously or
Lorfan 0.3-1.2 mg subcutaneously or intravenously every 15 minutes until normal
respiration pattern returns and there is
response to stimuli

— Do not give either Narcan or Nalline in cases
of Novrad (levoproxype) or Talwin (penta-
zocine) poisoning else symptoms may be
intensified. Nalline will act as a depressant
in absence of morphine or derivatives, so
be sure overdosage is of such a narcotic

— Avoid strong analeptics

2   If drug has been taken orally and patient is
    conscious, give activated charcoal (50 Gm/
    500 ml water shaken until all charcoal is
    wetted) and provoke vomiting (keep head
    down, prevent aspiration)

This may be administered and removed
through lavage tube. Repeat once

— Perform gastric lavage with a weak
solution 1-2000 of potassium permanganate
where available. Otherwise use tap water or
normal saline solution (100 ml-500 ml)

— Follow with magnesium sulfate cathartic

Lavage is useful even if delayed, as narcotics induce gastrointestinal spasm which may delay absorption

3 If drug has been injected, check its absorption by applying tourniquet to extremities. Release every 15 minutes. Use only enough pressure to occlude venous return. Apply ice pack to site of injection or immerse extremity in water (10°C) to slow capillary blood flow

4 Treat shock and coma conventionally

5 Supportive measures

— Keep patient warm

— Give conscious patients strong, black coffee to drink

— Administer adequate fluid intake

— Monitor fluid intake/output balance.

Narcotics

Phenothiazines and Related Drugs

Clinical Signs

Drowsiness
Disorientation
Dryness of mucosa
Blurred or double vision
Nasal congestion
Restlessness
Anxiety
Hyperactive tendon reflexes
Tachycardia
Extrapyramidal syndrome

Parkinsonism: tremors, various degrees of rigidity, motor retardation, excessive salivation

Dystonia and Dyskinesia: tics, perioral spasms, oculogyric crisis, tonic and myoclonic twitches of lateral and bilateral muscle group, drooling

Akathisia: motor restlessness, inability to keep still, compulsion to be on the move

Postural hypotension can be critical if severe, as it may be complicated by
    shock or coma
    cardiovascular insufficiency
    coronary occlusion (myocardial infarct)
    cardiac arrhythmias, ECG changes

Convulsions—tonic, clonic or startle seizures—appear late

Respiratory depression

Temperature regulation disturbances including:
    chills
    elevated temperature
    lowered temperature

Bladder or bowel paralysis

Potentially dangerous combinations (especially in large quantities)
    Alcohol
    Barbiturates
    Minor tranquilizers
    Narcotics

Phenothiazines and related drugs potentiate
    Atropine
    Phosphorus insecticides

Treatment

1   Maintain open airway

— Provide respiratory assistance if needed

2   Promote elimination of drug

— Induce vomiting if patient is conscious.

    (Usual techniques of producing vomiting
    may not work because of anti-vomiting
    action of phenothiazines)

- Use gastric aspiration and lavage. Most phenothiazines are water soluble and delay gastric emptying, so lavage is useful even hours after ingestion

- Leave solution of sodium sulfate in stomach as cathartic (30 Gm/250 ml water)

- **Diuresis using intravenous fluids**

  Slowly administer 100-250 ml 25% Mannitol intravenously

  Do not mix Mannitol in transfusion set. Red cell crenation and agglutination may occur

3 **Manage convulsions with short-acting barbiturates.** Inhalation anesthesia has been used in some cases to control seizures. When using barbiturates remember that their sedative effect is potentiated by phenothiazines. Avoid other depressant drugs

4 Treatment for extrapyramidal signs

- Parkinsonism can be treated with Akineton, Artane, Parsidol, Cogentin, Benadryl or other antiParkinsonian agent orally or intravenously

- Treat dyskinesia with an injection of 120 mg of sodium phenobarbital which may be repeated. Or use 0.5 Gm of caffeine sodium benzoate intravenously. It also may be repeated

5 Severe postural hypotension/shock/coma

- Elevate feet
- Maintain body warmth with blankets or heat cradles
- Use no external heat. It may aggravate shock or produce local damage

- Maintain blood volume with intravenous fluids

- Administer vasopressors: Levophed 0.2% solution, 4 ml/1000 ml of 5% dextrose. Or use Neo-Synephrine 10 mg/500 ml 5% dextrose in water or saline

- Do not give epinephrine or related compounds; action may be paradoxical. Maintain fluid and electrolyte balance

- Stimulants are of limited value and should be given cautiously

  Ritalin 10-50 mg 3 times daily, IV or IM. Or use dextroamphetamine 10 mg. Or administer caffeine sodium benzoate

- Phenothiazines lower convulsive threshold, so do not give convulsant stimulants such as Picrotoxin or Metrazol (pentylenetetrazol)

- Exchange transfusions have been recommended in children to remove protein bound drug in circulation

6 General supportive measures

- Maintain free airway

→

- Use suction to remove pharyngeal and nasal secretions
- Apply cold sponges and ice packs in hyperpyrexia (high temperature)
- Use blankets and heat cradles in hypothermia (lowered temperature)
- Record fluid intake and output

Special Notes

Severe hypotension may follow preoperative use of phenothiazines

This must be borne in mind if emergency calls for surgery

Patients who seem to be recovering from the overdosage may suddenly exhibit respiratory failure, cardiac arrhythmias or shock

Patient's progress must be watched until he is well out of CNS depression

Peritoneal dialysis and hemodialysis have not been found very effective.

Tricyclic Antidepressants

The signs and symptoms may be grouped as
follows

I   Atropine-like
II Neurological
III Cardiovascular

Atropine-like signs

Dry mouth
Mydriasis (dilated pupils)
Blurred vision
Sinus tachycardia (rapid heart, pulse beat);
    persistent, but, on the whole, benign
Ileus (bowel) paralysis
Bladder paralysis

Neurological signs

Coma vigil (light, arousable coma); may be
    interrupted by myoclonic convulsions and
    epileptic states. Coma recedes within 12
    hours. If coma is deep, suspect combinations
    of drugs
Respiratory depression: irregular, weak,
    rapid, stertorous (snorting) respirations
Ataxia (unsteadiness), atheroid and clonic
    movements
Agitation, delirium
Hyper-reflexive tendons
Extrapyramidal type of rigidity, e.g., cogwheel
Convulsions generally appear early during
    coma, are of few minutes duration, occur
    every 5 minutes, are mainly clonic, are
    highly characteristic
Disturbances of temperature regulation
Severe sweating, which may be of cardio-
    vascular origin
Hyperpyrexia (high fever) frequently is a
    cause of death

Cardiovascular signs

Cyanosis; rapid, weak pulse
Sinus tachycardia (rapid heart rate) is not
    serious by itself, but may be complicated
    by conduction disturbances of grave
    prognosis
Hypertension
    or
Hypotension
Shock
Conduction and rhythm disturbances are the
    chief differentiating characteristics of
    tricyclic overdosage

Major distinguishing overdosage features

1   Atrial fibrillation
2   Atrio-ventricular block
3   Intra-ventricular block
4   Ventricular flutter

→

ECG evidence of impaired conduction: QRS
interval equal to or greater than .12 second

Signs of congestive heart failure

Cardiovascular signs appear 30 minutes to
24 hours after ingestion of drug and with
treatment disappear 48 to 60 hours later

Potentially dangerous combinations

Sympathomimetics, e.g., epinephrine, etc.
Anticholinergics, e.g., atropine, antiParkinson
drugs, etc.
Monoamine Oxidase Inhibitors may result in
hyperpyretic crisis or severe convulsive
seizures
Vasopressors

Treatment

1   If cardiac complications and respiratory
depression are present, deal with them first

2   Elimination of drug

— Vomiting

— **Use gastric aspiration and lavage,** followed by
sodium sulfate catharsis (leave solution of
30 Gm in 250 ml water) in stomach. Intubate
unconscious patients with cuffed endotracheal
tube. Save aspirate and washings for
laboratory study

— **Continuous stomach lavage** with 10 to 20
liters of saline is recommended because of

Low plasma levels

High rate of drug secretion into stomach

Drug's atropinic effect which inhibits peristalsis

— **Elimination of tricyclics is essentially renal.** If
an inordinately large overdosage has been
taken, an artificial kidney may be useful in
eliminating the drug. Prolonged diuresis to
wash out possible second wave of metabolites
is useful

— Catheterize periodically. Remember there
may be bladder paralysis

— Peritoneal and hemodialysis have not been
found useful on the whole

3   Respiration

— Maintain open airway

— Use artificial respiration, oxygen where
necessary

— It has been suggested that in significant
overdosage with these drugs the patient should
be intubated with a cuffed endotracheal tube
prior to definite respiratory depression.
Should an emergency then arise, aid in
respiration can be quickly supplied

> — Guard tongue by inserting padded tongue depressor in mouth

— Control with any of the following

Diazepam (Valium) (IM 5-10 mg)

Short-acting barbiturates. Keep alert, however, to possible onset of respiratory depression

No barbiturates should be used if patient has also been on monoamine oxidase inhibitors

— Administer paraldehyde rectally, especially for children, since it does not depress respirations

— **Use succinylcholine only when strict control of patient ventilation is possible, preferably by an anesthetist**

5 Treatment for hypotension/shock should be aimed at supporting heart rate and stroke volume

— Start slow intravenous infusion of isotonic solutions

— Do not overhydrate. If there is heart damage, cardiac failure may ensue

— Administer plasma expanders

— Monitor electrolytes

— Do not use vasopressors

6 If hypertension is serious give phentolamine (Regitine) 5 mg

7 Cardiovascular problems

a. **Arrhythmias:** xylocaine (Lidocaine) or procainamide (Pronestyl) may be given intravenously. Electric shock may be necessary in persistent arrhythmias

b. **Conduction disorders:** intravenous infusion of 1/6 molar sodium lactate
Monitor ECG continuously for possible rapid changes in cardiac rhythm. Make provision for emergency defibrillation and resuscitation. Transvenous pacemaker for temporary pacing may be required

c. **If cardiac failure is imminent,** digitalize the patient rapidly via intravenous or intramuscular routes. Monitor and proceed very cautiously as medication may have additional toxic effect on myocardium

Do not digitalize if there are conduction defects or ventricular irritability. Instead, control with diuretics

d. **Cardiac arrest:** apply full resuscitative measures such as external cardiac massage, etc. Anticipate and avoid this possibility by placement of a temporary transvenous pacemaker

→

Tricyclic
Antidepressants

e. Maintain fluid/electrolyte and acid/base balance

Avoid Quinidine. It reduces speed of conduction

Avoid Epinephrine

8 Hyperpyrexia: apply cold sponges, ice packs and ice mattress (see Hyperpyrexia, p. 16)

9 Supportive care should include

— Systematic recording of vital signs

— Assistance of respiration by

positional changes
suctioning of mucous secretions
systematic recording of intake/output
quiet surroundings
catheterization as needed.

Cocaine

Clinical Signs

Restlessness, excitability
Euphoria, hallucinations
Dry mouth
Dilated pupils (mydriasis)
Increased reflexes
Chills or fever
Abdominal pain
Nausea, vomiting
Muscle spasms
Numbness
Rapid pulse initially; later, may be slow and weak
Pallor
Irregular, rapid respirations; later, shallow and slow
Convulsions of cerebral origin
Hypotension
Circulatory failure
Coma
Respiratory collapse

Treatment

1   Give water, milk or activated charcoal (50 Gm in 500 ml water) to induce vomiting

2   Remove by gastric lavage using solution of potassium permanganate 1:2000
Following lavage instill a saline cathartic (30 Gm sodium sulfate in 250 ml water)

3   If drug has been used on mucous membranes, wash membranes with tap water or normal saline solution

4   If drug has been injected, check absorption by applying tourniquet and ice bag at injection site

5   Convulsions
— Administer thiopental sodium 2.5% intravenously, slowly
— Or administer open-drop ether with minute-to-minute control
— Short-acting barbiturates also may be used
— Do not use morphine

6   Respiratory difficulties
— Give artificial respiration and oxygen as needed
— If convulsions interfere with respiration, succinylcholine 10-50 mg may be given intravenously, but artificial respiration must be administered concurrently

7   Supportive measures
— Keep patient warm by applying external heat to body; apply ice bag to head
— Keep patient in quiet surroundings
— Use padded restraints to prevent self-injury.

Lithium

Clinical Signs

Appear about 48 hours post-drug overdose
  ingestion
Confusion
Hypertonic or rigid muscles with hyperactive
  deep reflexes
Feeling of muscular weakness
Muscle tremor or fasciculation
Nausea, vomiting or abdominal pain
Diarrhea
Slurred speech
Thirst
Sudden hyperextension of the extremities often
  accompanied by grunts, gasping, and wide
  open eyes
Epileptic seizures
**Transitory neurological asymmetries simulating
  cerebral hemorrhage**
Coma with complete unresponsiveness
**Pulmonary complications such as atelectasis,
  pneumonia**

Treatment

1   Maintain open airway

2   Induce vomiting in conscious patients

3   Perform gastric lavage
— Use physiologic, saline or tap water
  (Potassium chloride 5-25 Gm orally has
  NOT been found effective in producing a
  decrease in blood lithium levels)

4   Regulate kidney function since lithium is
  excreted by the kidneys

5   Alkalinize urine

6   Force diuresis with fluids. Mannitol or urea
  may be used if necessary

7   Correct abnormalities in fluid and electrolyte
  balance

8   Take frequent blood pressure readings

9   Coma:
— Treat conventionally. Be alert to pulmonary
  complications while patient is in this state

— **Make frequent positional changes**

— **Keep X-ray surveillance of lungs**

10   Administer aminophyllin where necessary

11   Hemodialysis may be of use, but insufficient
  data on its use exists

12   General nursing care is of special importance
  in care of the comatose patient.

Lysergic Acid Diethylamide (L.S.D.)

Clinical Signs

Dilated pupils (mydriasis)
Blurred vision
Distortion of perception
Hearing acuity
Tremor, exaggerated reflexes
Fever
Relaxed, happy, frightened, or depressed mood
Mental dissociation, difficulties with simple
    problems
Time distortion, e.g., belief that numbers of years
    have gone by
Seeming psychotic personality disorders
Sometimes there are hallucinations; however,
    these occur less if subject is blindfolded and
    not at all if subject is blind

Special Notes

Lysergic Acid Diethylamide is:

    a psychotomimetic
    semi-synthetic
    derived from ergonovine

Treatment

1   Effect of drug lasts several hours depending
     on amount ingested

— Protect the individual from imprudent actions,
     self-injury, etc.

2   Give chlorpromazine, 50 mg IM every 3 hours
     until drug's effects subside

— Otherwise, treat symptomatically

— **Avoid reserpine since it heightens described
     symptoms**

3   Treatment generally is protective
     and symptomatic.

Marijuana and Hashish

Clinical Signs

(Effects become apparent rapidly if drug in form
of cigarette is inhaled; effects appear in
1/2 to 1 hour if drug is ingested)
Increase in pulse rate
Some increase in blood pressure
Dryness of mouth and throat
Nausea and vomiting
Hunger, desire for sweets
Congestion of conjunctiva at times
Frequency of urination
Ataxia, unsteady gait
Exhilaration
Disturbances of perception
Dreamy state; free flowing, disconnected ideas
Panic states, hallucinations, fear of death may
occur with large doses
Stupor, coma, and/or respiratory depression

Treatment

1   Main treatment is protective and symptomatic

2   Treat as for a physiological depression by
maintaining

— open airway

— adequate oxygen intake and carbon dioxide
removal

— blood pressure at adequate levels

3   If drug has been ingested, attempt its
elimination in conscious patients by vomiting

— If patient is unconscious, lavage after carefully placing endotracheal tube. Catharsis
should be induced by leaving a solution of
30 Gm sodium sulfate in 250 ml water in
stomach after lavage

4   Analeptics such as caffeine, amphetamine,
megimide (Bemegride) are rarely indicated.
They may be tried, but not if there is severe
respiratory depression

5   **Be alert to complications which can result from
stimulant therapy, i.e., arrhythmias,
convulsions, cardiac failure, etc.**

Mescaline

Clinical Signs

Headache
Dilated pupils (mydriasis)
Nausea and vomiting
Hallucinations

Treatment

1   Provoke emesis

2   Perform gastric lavage. Leave saline
solution of sodium sulfate 30 Gm (1 oz)
in 250 ml (glass) of water in stomach
as cathartic

3   Treat symptomatically.

Ritalin

Clinical Signs

Dry mucous membranes
Vomiting
Tremors, agitation
Muscle twitching, hyperreflexia
Confusion, euphoria
Dilated pupils (mydriasis)
Headache
Hallucinations
Fever
Hypertension
Palpitation, tachycardia, cardiac arrhythmias

Treatment

1   Treat symptomatically

2   In severe intoxication administer carefully
titrated dosage of short-acting barbiturate
before gastric lavage

—   Dialysis and hemodialysis have not been
found useful.

Book's Color Code	Brand Name N D C Numbers	Generic/ Chemical Name	Classification	Use	Street Name(s)	Manufacturer	Packaging
	Adipex Ty-Med 93-0004 93-0032	methamphet- amine HCl amobarbital	amphetamine & barbiturate	stimulation/ sedation	Speedballs	Lemmon	Tablets (NDC93-0004) and capsules (NDC93-0032): Bottles of 100 & 1000 **Notes:** There may be excessive stimulation or excessive depression See Amphetamine or Barbiturate Sections If there is excessive stimulation, do not use a barbiturate in treatment Currently withdrawn from market
	Akineton 44-0120 44-0110	biperiden HCl	antiParkinson	antiParkinson		Knoll	Tablets (NDC44-0120): 2 mg—round—white—indented with triangle—bisected on obverse side—bottles of 100 & 1000 Sterile solution (NDC44-0110): ampules—IM, IV—5 mg/ml—10 1 ml ampules/box
	Alurate 4-1000 4-1001	aprobarbital	barbiturate	sedative & hypnotic	Barbs, Downers, Goofballs	Roche	Elixir (NDC4-1000): red—40 mg/teaspoon in bottles of 16 oz and one gallon Elixir Verdum (NDC4-1001): green—40 mg/teaspoon in bottles of 16 oz
	Amytal 2-OT40 2-OT56 2-OT37 2-OT32 2-OX36 2-OX41	amobarbital	barbiturate	sedative	Downers, Rainbows, Barbs, Goofballs, Blue Angels, Blue Devils, Blue Heavens	Lilly	Capsule-shaped scored tablets: 15 mg (1/4 gr) (NDC2-OT40)—light green—bottles of 100 & 500 30 mg (1/2 gr) (NDC2-OT56)—yellow—bottles of 100, 1000, 5000 50 mg (3/4 gr) (NDC2-OT37)—orange—bottles of 100, 500, 5000 100 mg (1½ gr) (NDC2-OT32)—pink—bottles of 100 & 500 All impressed with name Lilly & NDC number Elixir #225 (NDC2-OX36): 440 mg/100 ml (2 gr/fl oz) in pint bottles Elixir #237 (NDC2-OX41): 880 mg/100 ml (4 gr/fl oz) in pint & gallon bottles

Name / Code	Generic	Class	Action	Street names	Manufacturer	Supply

Amytal Sodium
2-OF23
2-OF33
	sodium amobarbital	barbiturate	sedative	Blue Devils,
				Blue Angels,
				Blue Clouds,
				Bluebirds,
				Blue Heavens,
				Downers
					Lilly	Capsules: 65 mg (1 gr) (NDC2-OF23)—blue—imprinted Lilly F23—
						   bottles of 100, 500, 5000
						   200 mg (3 gr) (NDC2-OF33)—blue—imprinted Lilly F33—bottles of 100, 500
						Suppositories: 200 mg (3 gr)—packages of 10
						Ampules: dry powder in amounts to deliver varying strengths when
						   dissolved—65 mg (1 gr), 130 mg (2 gr), 260 mg (4 gr), 500 mg (7½ gr)

Artane
5-4434
5-4436
5-4438
5-4440
	trihexyphenidyl HCl	antiParkinson	antiParkinson		Lederle	Tablets: white—scored—2 mg (NDC5-4434) & 5 mg (NDC5-4436) each—
						   bottles of 100, 1000, 5000
						Sequels (NDC5-4438): blue—5 mg—bottles of 30 & 500
						Elixir (NDC5-4440): lime colored—mint flavored—2 mg/5 ml—
						   bottles of 16 fl oz

Atarax
49-5600
49-5610
49-5620
49-5630
49-5590
49-5530
49-5540
49-5560
49-5570
49-5580
	hydroxyzine HCl	antihistamine	sedative &
			anxiolytic
					Roerig	Coated tablets: 10 mg (NDC49-5600)—orange—bottles of 100 & 500
						   25 mg (NDC49-5610)—green—bottles of 100 & 500
						   50 mg (NDC49-5620)—yellow—bottles of 100 & 500
						   100 mg (NDC49-5630)—red—bottles of 100
						Syrup (NDC49-5590): pale yellow—vanilla flavor—
						   10 mg/teaspoon (5 ml)—supplied in 1 pint bottles
						Sterile solutions: IM—25 mg/ml (NDC49-5530)
						   IM—50 mg/ml (NDC49-5540)
						   Isoject, IM—25 mg/ml (NDC49-5560)
						   Isoject, IM—50 mg/ml (NDC49-5570)
						   Isoject, IM—100 mg/ml (NDC49-5580)

Aventyl
2-OH17
2-OH19
2-OX68
	nortriptyline HCl	tricyclic	anti-
			depressant
					Lilly	Capsules: 10 mg (NDC2-OH17) 25 mg (NDC2-OH19)
						   Both strengths have white opaque body, yellow opaque cap, with Lilly &
						   NDC imprint on each half, & come in bottles of 100 & 500 and in 10 strips
						   of 10 individually labeled blisters each containing one capsule
						Clarification: Liquid (NDC2-OX68): colorless—odorless—tasteless—
						   10 mg/5 ml in pint bottles

Book's Color Code	Brand Name NDC Numbers	Generic/ Chemical Name	Classification	Use	Street Name(s)	Manufacturer	Packaging
	Bancaps 291-1005 291-1010	acetaminophen/ salicylamide/ butabarbital	antianxiety	analgesic & mild sedative		Westerfield	Bancaps Capsule (NDC291-1005): acetaminophen 300 mg, salicylamide 200 mg, butabarbital sodium 10 mg—bottles of 100 & 500 capsules Also Bancaps-C Capsule (NDC291-1010): Contains formula in Bancaps (above) plus 30 mg (1/2 gr) Codeine phosphate Supplied in bottles of 40 & 100 capsules **Note:** Closely observe renal function
	Benadryl 71-0373 71-0471 71-1090 71-1235 71-1219 71-1028 71-1149 71-1402 71-1257 71-1406	diphenhydra- mine HCl	antihistamine	antihistamine & sedative		Parke Davis	Kapseals (NDC71-0373): light red capsule, white center band—contains 50 mg diphenhydramine HCl—marked P-D 373 Capsules (NDC71-0471): white body, red cap—contains 25 mg diphenhydramine HCl—marked P-D 471 Both strengths come in bottles of 100 & 1000 Cream - 2% (NDC71-1090) Elixir (NDC71-1235): oral—12.5 mg/5 ml—in 4 oz, 16 oz, 1 gal, 5 ml unit-dose bottles Powder (NDC71-1219): bulk—oral—1/2 oz vial Sterile solutions: steri-vial—parenteral use—10 mg/ml—10 ml (NDC71-1028), 30 ml (NDC71-1149) vials Sterile solution for parenteral use (NDC71-1402)—50 mg/ml in 10 ml steri-vials Sterile solution for parenteral use (NDC71-1257)—50 mg/ml—1 cc ampules Sterile solution (NDC71-1406): steri-dose syringe for parenteral use— 50 mg/ml in boxes of 10 **Notes:** Stimulants should not be used in treatment Use only short-acting barbiturate in small doses if convulsions occur

Benzedrine 7-OA91 7-OA92 7-OA90	amphetamine sulfate	amphetamine	anorectic & stimulant	A, Bennies, Ups or Uppers, Peaches, Hearts, Jolly Beans, Bombitas, Cartwheels, Lid Proppers, Thrusters, Roses, Fives (for 5 mg tablets), Forwards, Pep Pills	Smith, Kline & French	Tablets: 5 mg (NDC7-OA91), 10 mg (NDC7-OA92)—two sizes—peach color—triangular—scored—bottles of 100—impressed A91, A92 Spansules (taper end capsules) (NDC7-OA90): 15 mg amphetamine sulfate—clear body, cap with SKF imprint & marked A90—bottles of 50 **Note:** In overdosage with "Spansules" bear in mind that medication is released gradually. Therapy should be continued for as long as overdosage symptoms are present
Buticaps 45-0060 45-0061 45-0062 45-0063	sodium butabarbital	barbiturate	sedative	Downs, Barbs, Goofballs	McNeil	Capsules: 15 mg (1/4 gr) (NDC45-0060)—lavender and white 30 mg (1/2 gr) (NDC45-0061)—green and white 50 mg (3/4 gr) (NDC45-0062)—orange and white 100 mg (1½ gr) (NDC45-0063)—pink and white McNeil imprint on body & cap of all capsules—All in bottles of 100
Butisol Sodium 45-0112 45-0113 45-0114 45-0115 45-0116 45-0117 45-0110	sodium butabarbital	barbiturate	sedative	Barbs, Downers, Goofballs	McNeil	Tablets: 15 mg (1/4 gr) (NDC45-0112)—lavender 30 mg (1/2 gr) (NDC45-0113)—green 50 mg (3/4 gr) (NDC45-0114)—orange 100 mg (1½ gr) (NDC45-0115)—pink All scored—engraved McNeil—not coated Tablets R-A (repeat action): 30 mg (1/2 gr) (NDC45-0116)—coated white, imprinted in lavender 60 mg (1 gr) (NDC45-0117)—coated white, imprinted green Elixir (NDC45-0110): green—alcohol 7%—30 mg/5 ml

Book's Color Code	Brand Name N D C Numbers	Generic/ Chemical Name	Classification	Use	Street Name(s)	Manufacturer	Packaging
	Chloral Hydrate	chloral hydrate	barbiturate-like	sedative & hypnotic	Knock-out Drops, Mickey Finn (liquid chloral hydrate and alcohol), Peter, Joy Juice	Many manufac-turers (36)	This drug is packaged by 36 manufacturers under generic name of chloral hydrate in capsules and tablets for oral use and also as an elixir or syrup, in crystals or bulk, & in suppositories **Notes:** See **Felsules, Kessodrate Capsules, Noctec** Patients suffer gastric distress Quick circulatory collapse may occur
	Cocaine 2-OY14	from Erythroxylon Coca	miscellaneous	stimulant	Coke, Snow, C, or Big C, Bernice, Bernies, Corrine, Flake, Girl, Happy Dust, Gold Dust, Star Dust, Her, Heaven Dust, Burese	Lilly	Soluble tablets (Solvets) (NDC2-OY14)—topical—135 mg—100 in bottle **Notes:** Do not use **Morphine** in treatment of overdosage Sniffed or injected
	Codeine There are 48 NDCs	methylmorphine	narcotic	narcotic depressant	Turps (for Elixir of Terpin Hydrate with Codeine), School Boys	Several manufacturers including American Pharmaceutical Co., Blue Line, Ciba, Kirkman, Knoll, Lilly, Noyes, Premo, Stanley Drug, USV Pharmaceutical Co., Vitarine, Wyeth	Oral tablets Tablets for solution (parenteral use) Sterile solutions for injection: SC & IM Ingredient in many cough preparations **Notes:** Antidote: **Nalline** (5-10 mg IM or IV) Convulsions a likely complication Avoid strong analeptics

	Cogentin 6-0021 6-0635 6-0060 6-3275	benztropine mesylate	antiParkinson	antiParkinson	Merck Sharp & Dohme	Tablets: 0.5 mg (NDC6-0021)—white—flat—round—scored on 1 side—bottles of 100 1.0 mg (NDC6-0635)—white—oval shaped—scored on 1 side—bottles of 100 2.0 mg (NDC6-0060)—white—flat—round—quarter-sected on 1 side— bottles of 100 & 1000 All tablets uncoated, engraved with MSD & NDC number Injection (NDC6-3275): 1 mg/ml in 2 ml ampules
	Compazine 7-OC66 7-OC67 7-OC69 7-OC44 7-OC46 7-OC47 7-OC49 7-OC63 7-OC42 7-OC43 7-OC60 7-OC61 7-OC62	prochlorper-azine	phenothiazine	major tranquilizer	Smith, Kline & French	Tablets: 5 mg (NDC7-OC66) 10 mg (NDC7-OC67) 25 mg (NDC7-OC69) All are chartreuse—coated—SKF & dosage imprinted on each— bottles of 100 & 1000—marked C66, C67, C69 respectively Capsules: 10 mg (NDC7-OC44)—SKF & one dot imprinted—marked C44 15 mg (NDC7-OC46)—SKF & two dots imprinted—marked C46 30 mg (NDC7-OC47)—SKF & three dots imprinted—marked C47 75 mg (NDC7-OC49)—SKF & four dots imprinted—marked C49 All are yellow & blue spansules Syrup (NDC7-OC63)—dark amber—bitter tasting—fruit fragrance— 5 mg/5 ml in 4 oz bottles Concentrate (NDC7-OC41): 10 mg/ml in 4 oz bottles, 36 bottles in carton Injection, IM, IV (NDC7-OC42 & 7-OC43)—5 mg/ml (2 ml ampule)—boxes of 6, 100, 500—multiple-dose 10 ml vials—boxes of 1, 20, 100 Suppositories: 2.5 mg (NDC7-OC60)—single yellow stripe, dosage imprinted 5 mg (NDC7-OC61)—double yellow stripe, dosage imprinted 25 mg (NDC7-OC62)—yellow band with dosage, ADULT imprinted
	Dartal 14-0201 14-0211	thiopropazate HCl	phenothiazine	major tranquilizer	Searle	Tablets: 5 mg (NDC14-0201)—coated—white 10 mg (NDC14-0211)—coated—peach color In bottles of 50 & 100

Book's Color Code	Brand Name N D C Numbers	Generic/ Chemical Name	Classification	Use	Street Name(s)	Manufacturer	Packaging
	Darvon 2-OH02 2-OH03 2-OH04 2-OH05 2-OH06 2-OH11 2-OC53 2-OC54	propoxy- phene HCl	narcotic	analgesic	Dummies	Lilly	Darvon (NDC2-OH02 & 2-OH03) Capsules: 32 mg (Code H02) & 65 mg (Code H03); both opaque light pink Darvon Compound (Code H05) (NDC2-OH05) Capsules: 32 mg propoxyphene HCl, 227 mg aspirin, 162 mg phenacetin, 32.4 mg caffeine Light pink opaque body, light grey opaque cap Darvon Compound 65 (Code H06) (NDC2-OH06) Capsules: 65 mg propoxyphene HCl, 227 mg aspirin, 162 mg phenacetin, 32.4 mg caffeine Light red opaque body, light grey opaque cap Darvon with ASA (Code H04) (NDC2-OH04) Capsules: 65 mg propoxyphene HCl, 325 mg aspirin Red opaque body, pink opaque cap All the capsules above bear Lilly imprint, identifying code number All in bottles of 100 & 500, in 10 strips of 10 blisters with one labeled capsule each, & in strip packages of individually sealed capsules Darvo-Tran (Code H11) (NDC2-OH11) Capsules: 32 mg propoxyphene HCl, 325 mg aspirin, 150 mg phenaglycodol Light pink opaque body, maroon opaque cap—bottles of 100 & 500 Darvon-N (propoxyphene napsylate) (NDC2-OC53) Tablets: 100 mg—specially coated—buff color—bottles of 100 & 500 & 10 strips of 10 individually labeled blisters with 1 tablet Suspension: 50 mg/5 ml in bottles of 16 fl oz Darvon-N with ASA (propoxyphene napsylate 100 mg with aspirin 325 mg) (NDC2-OC54) Tablets: Specially coated—orange—bottles of 100 & 500, 10 strips of 10 individually labeled blisters each containing 1 tablet

Demerol
See
Packaging

Demerol	meperidine HCl	narcotic	analgesic, spasmolytic, sedative	Breon Winthrop

Breon

Demerol
  Sterile solutions: 50 mg/ml—IM, IV, SC—(NDC57-OD21)
    100 mg/ml—IM, IV, SC—(NDC57-OD22)
  Tablets: 50 mg (NDC57-OD25)
Demerol APAP (NDC57-OD31)
  Tablets: meperidine HCl 50 mg & acetaminophen 300 mg—round—
    pink & red mottled
Demerol Compound (NDC57-OD29)
  Tablets: meperidine HCl 25 mg, hydrocodone bitartrate 5 mg,
    acetaminophen 150 mg—stratified in three layers of pink,
    white (center), green

Winthrop

Tablets: 50 mg—(NDC24-OD35)—white—bottles of 100, 250, 500, 1000
  100 mg—(NDC24-OD37)—white—bottles of 100 & 500
  All have Winthrop engraved on outer edge
Elixir: 50 mg/teaspoon—(NDC24-OD33)—nonalcoholic—banana flavor—
  bottles of 16 fl oz
For parenteral use
5% solution (50 mg/ml):
  Vials of 10 & 30 mg
  Ampules of 0.5 ml (25 mg), 1 ml (50 mg)—in boxes of 25 & 100;
    1.5 ml (75 mg), 2 ml (100 mg)—boxes of 5, 25, 100
  Cartridges of 1 ml (50 mg)—disposable plastic syringe—boxes of 10;
    1 ml (50 mg) in 2 ml—disposable plastic syringe—boxes of 10
7.5% solution (75 mg/ml):
  Cartridges of 1 ml in disposable syringe—boxes of 10;
    1 ml in 2 ml disposable plastic syringe—boxes of 10
10% solution (100 mg/ml):
  Vials of 20 ml
  Ampules of 1 ml (100 mg), boxes of 25, 100
  Cartridges of 1 ml (100 mg) in disposable plastic syringe—boxes of 10;
    1 ml (100 mg) in 2 ml disposable plastic syringe—boxes of 10
Note: Antidote: Nalorphine or levallorphan. See package insert for
instructions on use
Demerol is potentiated by MAOIs.

Book's Color Code	Brand Name N D C Numbers	Generic/ Chemical Name	Classification	Use	Street Name(s)	Manufacturer	Packaging
	Desbutal 74-3991 74-6806 74-6814	methamphet-amine HCl & sodium pentobarbital	amphetamine & barbiturate	anorectic & mood elevating	Speedballs, Grads, Yellow BAMs (15 mg only), Greenies (capsules)	Abbott	Capsule (NDC74-3991): green—containing 5 mg methamphetamine HCl & 30 mg sodium pentobarbital—imprinted with Abbott trademark & name Abbott—bottles of 100, 1000 Gradumet tablets: Orange & blue—10 mg methamphetamine HCl & 60 mg sodium pentobarbital (NDC74-6806) Yellow & blue—15 mg methamphetamine HCl & 90 mg sodium pentobarbital (NDC74-6814) Both tablets engraved with Abbott trademark, in bottles of 100 & 500
		Notes: In treating overdosage of **Desbutal** it has been reported that usually the effect of the barbiturate predominates. The Gradumet matrix is insoluble in water, so consider provoking emesis first. When overdose is with the capsules, lavage as soon as possible					There may be excessive stimulation or excessive depression See Amphetamine or Barbiturate Sections If there is excessive stimulation do not use a barbiturate in treatment Currently withdrawn from market
	Desoxy-ephedrine	desoxy-ephedrine HCl (methamphet-amine HCl)	amphetamine	mood elevating	Crystal, Speed, Meth, Bombitas, Uppers		Following manufacturers supply this drug under its generic name: Atlas Pharmaceutical: Solution—20 mg/1cc ampules Harvey: Tablets—5 mg & 10 mg—both in bottles of 1000 Lanpar: Tablets—5 mg—bottles of 1000 Pehurst Pharmacal: Parenteral solution—20 mg/cc in 30 cc vials Robinson: Powder—1 oz containers Tablets—5 mg—bottles of 100 & 1000 Truxton, C.O.: Parenteral solutions—20 mg/cc in 30 cc vials Tablets—5 mg & 10 mg—both in bottles of 1000 **Notes:** See **Methamphetamine HCl** This drug now is known as Methamphetamine HCl, but still is listed in many catalogs and sold under the names (d)-desoxyephedrine and/or desoxyephedrine HCl

Desoxyn 74-3488 74-3377 74-6941 74-6948 74-6959	methamphet-amine HCl	amphetamine	anorectic & mood elevating	Splash, Wakeups, Rippers, Meth, Leapers, Lid-poppers, Forwards, Crank, Copilot, Speed, Grads, Crystal, Pep Pills, Yellow BAMs (15 mg only), Bombitas, Uppers	Abbott	Tablets: 2.5 mg (NDC74-3488)—white—bottles of 100 5.0 mg (NDC74-3377)—white—bottles of 100 & 1000 Gradumet, uncoated tablets: 5 mg (NDC74-6941)—white—bottles of 100 10 mg (NDC74-6948)—orange—bottles of 100 15 mg (NDC74-6959)—yellow—bottles of 100 & 500 Gradumet tablets engraved with Abbott trademark
Dexamyl 7-0093 7-0091 7-0092 7-0090	dextro-amphetamine/amobarbital	amphetamine & barbiturate	anorectic & stimulant	Dexies, Dex, Speedballs, Christmas Trees, (Purple Hearts or French Blues for British analogue Drinamyl—a purple tablet)	Smith, Kline & French	Tablet (NDC7-0093): green—scored—uncoated—triangular—containing 5 mg dextroamphetamine sulfate—32 mg (1/2 gr) amobarbital—engraved SKF and 093—bottles of 100 & 1000 Spansule: taper end capsule—clear with green cap—#1 & #2 imprinted SKF & code in white—bottles of 50 & 500 (#1) 10 mg dextroamphetamine sulfate & 65 mg (1 gr) amobarbital (NDC7-0091) (#2) 15 mg dextroamphetamine sulfate & 100 mg (1½ gr) amobarbital (NDC7-0092) Elixir (NDC7-0090): 5 ml/teaspoon containing 5 mg dextroamphetamine sulfate & 32 mg amobarbital—bottles of 16 fl oz **Notes:** In overdosage there may be excessive sedation or excessive stimulation. Treat symptomatically If a sedative is needed because of excessive stimulation, do not use a barbiturate See Amphetamine or Barbiturate Sections Currently withdrawn from market

Book's Color Code	Brand Name N D C Numbers	Generic/ Chemical Name	Classification	Use	Street Name(s)	Manufacturer	Packaging
	Dexedrine 7-OE19 7-OE11 7-OE12 7-OE13 7-OE14	dextro-amphetamine sulfate	amphetamine	anorectic & stimulant	A, Dexies, Oranges, Speed, Splash, Crank, Copilots, Lid-poppers, Lid-proppers, Pep Pills, Truckdrivers, Ups or Uppers, Wakeups, Hearts, Cartwheels, Xmas Trees, Thrusters, Sparkle Plenties, Brownies	Smith, Kline & French	Tablets (NDC7-OE19): 5 mg—peach color—triangular—scored—engraved SKF, E19—uncoated—bottles of 100 & 1000 Elixir (NDC7-OE11): 5 mg/teaspoon—bottles of 16 fl oz Spansule capsules (taper end): 5 mg (NDC7-OE12)—SKF imprint—bottles of 50 10 mg (NDC7-OE13)—SKF & one dot imprinted 15 mg (NDC7-OE14)—SKF & two dots imprinted Both 10 & 15 mg capsules in bottles of 50 & 500
	Dilaudid 44-1021 44-1022 44-1023 44-1024 44-1011 44-1012 44-1013 44-1014 44-1060 44-1053 44-1080 44-1040	hydro-morphone HCl	narcotic	narcotic, analgesic	Little D	Knoll	Tablets: 1 mg (NDC44-1021), 2 mg (NDC44-1022), 3 mg (NDC44-1023), 4 mg (NDC44-1024)—bottles of 100 Ampules: 1 mg/ml (NDC44-1011), 2 mg/ml (NDC44-1012), 3 mg/ml (NDC44-1013), 4 mg/ml (NDC44-1014)—boxes of 10, 2 mg/cc—boxes of 25—SC, IM, IV Sterile solutions: 1 mg/ml in 10 & 20 ml vials 2 mg/ml in 10 & 20 ml vials 3 mg/ml in 10 & 20 ml vials 4 mg/ml in 10 & 20 ml vials **Dilaudid Sulfate** (NDC44-1060): 2 mg/ml—multiple dose vials—SC, IM, IV Suppositories (NDC44-1053): 3 mg—boxes of 6 Tablet: misc. 30 mg Syrup (cough) (NDC44-1080): reddish-orange—peach flavored—pint bottles **Note:** Antidotes: **Nalline** or **Lorfan**

Disipal 89-0161	orphenadrine HCl	antihistamine	antiParkinson	Riker	Tablets (NDC89-0161): 50 mg—green—engraved Riker—bottles of 100 & 500
Dolophine HCl 2-OJ64 2-OJ72 2-OY30 2-OP82 2-OP87	methadone HCl	narcotic	narcotic, analgesic	Dolls, Dollies	Lilly	Tablets: 5 mg (NDC2-OJ64)—bottles of 100 & 1000 10 mg (NDC2-OJ72)—bottles of 100 Syrup (NDC2-OY30): 10 mg/30 ml—pint & gallon bottles Sterile solution for SC and IM use (NDC2-OP82 & 2-OP87)—10 mg/ml—20 cc vial & in 1 ml ampules **Note:** See **Methadone**
Doriden 83-0027 83-0114 83-0079 83-0070	glutethimide	barbiturate-like	sedative & anxiolytic	"D"	USV Pharmaceutical	Tablets: 0.125 Gm (NDC83-0027)—bottles of 100 0.25 Gm (NDC83-0114)—bottles of 100 & 1000 0.5 Gm (NDC83-0079)—bottles of 100, 500, 1000 All are white—.25 Gm & .5 Gm are scored—engraved USV—strip dispensers of 100 Capsules (NDC83-0070): 0.5 Gm—blue & white—USV imprinted in white—bottles of 100 **Notes:** Do not provoke vomiting; it could result in sudden cessation of respiration. Patients suffering from large overdoses may have to be intubated as a precautionary measure Hypotension is common: watch for circulatory shock
Elavil 6-0023 6-0045 6-0102 6-3286	amitriptyline HCl	tricyclic	anti-depressant	Merck Sharp & Dohme	Coated tablets: 10 mg (NDC6-0023)—blue—round 25 mg (NDC6-0045)—yellow—round Both in bottles of 100, 1000, 5000 50 mg (NDC6-0102)—beige—round—bottles of 100 & 1000 All tablets are imprinted MSD & with corresponding NDC Solution (NDC6-3286): 10 cc vials—10 mg/ml for injection

Book's Color Code	Brand Name N D C Numbers	Generic/ Chemical Name	Classification	Use	Street Name(s)	Manufacturer	Packaging
	Equanil 8-0002 8-0001 8-0044 8-0033 8-0230	meprobamate	antianxiety	sedative & anxiolytic	Downers	Wyeth	Tablets: 200 mg (NDC8-0002)—five sided—boxes of 50, 100, 500 & 1000 400 mg (NDC8-0001)—round—strip pack boxes of 25 & 100 Both tablets with Wyeth trademark W—uncoated—white—scored Capsule (NDC8-0044): clear and red—continuous-release capsule— 400 mg—bottles of 50 Wyseals (NDC8-0033): yellow coated tablet—400 mg—bottles of 50 & 500 Suspension (NDC8-0230): oral—200 mg/5cc **Note:** Patients may present varied clinical syndromes including chills, fever, peripheral edema, possibly convulsions, vasomotor and respiratory collapse, coma, shock, cardiac arrest See **Meprobamate**
	Eskabarb 7-OH74 7-OH76	phenobarbital	barbiturate	sedative	Phenos, Phennies, Downers, Goofballs, Barbs	Smith, Kline & French	Capsules: 1 gr (65 mg) (NDC7-OH74)—1 white dot on cap 1½ gr (97 mg) (NDC7-OH76)—2 white dots on cap Both are Spansules with SKF & appropriate NDC imprinted—clear body, blue cap—bottles of 50
	Eskalith 7-OJ07	lithium carbonate	miscellaneous	anti-depressant		Smith, Kline & French	Capsule (NDC7-OJ07): 300 mg—yellow & grey—imprinted SKF & J07— bottles of 100 and 1000
	Eskaphen B 7-OJ20 7-OJ19	phenobarbital & thiamin chloride	barbiturate	sedative	Phennies, Barbs, Goofers	Smith, Kline & French	Tablet (NDC7-OJ20): uncoated—round—peach color—engraved SKF J20—contains 1/4 gr phenobarbital (16 mg)—bottles of 50 Elixir (NDC7-OJ19): 1/4 gr/teaspoon—16 fl oz bottle

Name / Code	Generic	Class	Action	Street Names	Manufacturer	Description
Etrafon 85-OANA 85-OANC 85-OANB 85-OANE	perphenazine & amitriptyline HCl	phenothiazine & tricyclic	Both as tranquilizer & anti-depressant		Schering	Etrafon (2-10) (NDC85-OANA) 2 mg perphenazine & 10 mg amitriptyline HCl: yellow—imprinted with black Schering trademark & letters ANA Etrafon (2-25) (NDC85-OANC) 2 mg perphenazine & 25 mg amitriptyline HCl: pink—imprinted with brown Schering trademark & letters ANC Etrafon A (4-10) (NDC85-OANB) 4 mg perphenazine & 10 mg amitriptyline HCl: orange—imprinted with black Schering trademark & letters ANB Etrafon Forte (4-25) (NDC85-OANE) 4 mg perphenazine & 25 mg amitriptyline HCl: red—imprinted with blue Schering trademark & letters ANE All above are sugarcoated tablets supplied in bottles of 60 & 250 and also in boxes of 100 containing 10 strips of 10 tablets each for unit dose dispensing **Note:** See **Triavil**
Felsules 237-0400 237-0405 237-0410	chloral hydrate	barbiturate-like	sedative & hypnotic	Knock-out Drops, Mickey Finn (with alcohol), Joy Juice	Fellows Medical Manufac-turing	Capsules: 3¾ gr (0.25 Gm) (NDC237-0400)—blue & white—bottles of 100 & 500 7½ gr (0.5 Gm) (NDC237-0405)—blue—bottles of 50, 100, 250 15 gr (1 Gm) (NDC237-0410)—yellow—bottles of 30 & 100 **Notes:** Patients suffer gastric distress Quick circulatory collapse may occur
Halabar 86-0130	mephenesin & butabarbital	barbiturate	sedative & anxiolytic	Barbs, Goofballs	Carnrick	Tablets (NDC86-0130): 300 mg mephenesin & 16 mg butabarbital—bottles of 100
Haldol 45-0240 45-0241 45-0242 45-0245 45-0250	haloperidol	phenothiazine & related drugs	major tranquilizer		McNeil	Tablets: 0.5 mg (NDC45-0240)—white—scored—engraved 1/2 1.0 mg (NDC45-0241)—yellow—scored—engraved 1 2.0 mg (NDC45-0242)—pink—scored—engraved 2 5.0 mg (NDC45-0245)—green—scored—engraved 5 Bottles of 100, 1000, 5000; also bottle/box of 50 x 100 tablets Solution (NDC45-0250): Concentrate Haldol—2 mg/ml—colorless—odorless—tasteless—bottles of 15 ml and 120 ml **Note:** In treatment of overdosage with **Haldol, do not use epinephrine**

Book's Color Code	Brand Name N D C Numbers	Generic/ Chemical Name	Classification	Use	Street Name(s)	Manufacturer	Packaging
	Hashish Illegal	cannabis sativa	miscellaneous	halluci- nogenic	Bhang, Hash, Gram (for cube of hashish), Keif, Charas, Black Russian	**Illegal**	**Illegal** **Note:** Smoked or taken orally
	Heroin Illegal	diacetyl- morphine	narcotic	narcotic, analgesic, CNS depressant	H, Horse, Skag (Scag), Smak (Smack), Junk, Scat, Lemonade (poor heroin), Him, Boy, Doojee (Duji), Harry, Stuff, White Stuff, Shit, The White Lady, Tecata, Henry, Dogie	**Illegal in U.S.A.**	**Illegal** **Note: Heroin** is either sniffed, injected, or added to **Marijuana** and smoked
	Kemadrin 81-0602 81-0604	procyclidine HCl	antiParkinson	antiParkinson		Burroughs Wellcome	Tablets: 2 mg (NDC81-0602)—code imprinted F4B—bottles of 100 & 1000 5 mg (NDC81-0604)—bottles of 100, 1000, 5000
	Kesso- Bamate 22-0734 22-0570	meprobamate	antianxiety	sedative & anxiolytic	Downers	McKesson	Tablets: 200 mg (NDC22-0734) 400 mg (NDC22-0570) Both are round—white—scored McK—in bottles of 100 & 1000 **Note:** Overdosage may cause chills, fever, peripheral edema, possibly convulsions, vasomotor and respiratory collapse, coma, shock, cardiac arrest See **Meprobamate**

Kessodrate Capsules 22-0966 22-0967 22-0122	chloral hydrate	barbiturate-like	sedative & hypnotic	Knock-out Drops, Mickey Finn (with alcohol), Joy Juice	McKesson	Capsules: 250 mg (NDC22-0966) 500 mg (NDC22-0967) Both have rust color—"McKesson" imprinted—in bottles of 100 Syrup (NDC22-0122): 500 mg/5 ml—bottles of 16 fl oz & 1 gallon **Note:** Patients may suffer gastric distress; quick circulatory collapse may occur
Librax 4-0007	chlordiaze-poxide HCl & clidinium bromide	antianxiety	sedative & anxiolytic	Downers	Roche	Capsules (NDC4-0007): Green—5 mg chlordiazepoxide hydrochloride & 2.5 mg clidinium bromide—ROCHE and code 7 imprinted on each half—bottles of 100 & 500
Libritabs 4-0013 4-0014 4-0015	chlor-diazepoxide	antianxiety	sedative & anxiolytic		Roche	Tablets: 5 mg (NDC4-0013)—blue-green—13 imprinted 10 mg (NDC4-0014)—blue-green—14 imprinted 25 mg (NDC4-0015)—blue-green—15 imprinted All in bottles of 100 & 500
Librium 4-0001 4-0002 4-0003 4-1912	chlordiazepox-ide HCl	antianxiety	sedative & anxiolytic	Downers	Roche	Capsules: 5 mg (NDC4-0001)—green & yellow—ROCHE & 1 imprinted on each half 10 mg (NDC4-0002)—green & black—ROCHE & 2 imprinted on each half 25 mg (NDC4-0003)—green & white—ROCHE & 3 imprinted on each half All strengths in bottles of 100 & 500 and in Tel-E-Dose packages of 1000 Injection (NDC4-1912): Duplex package containing material for preparation of ampule of 100 mg/2 ml
Lithane 49-5660	lithium carbonate	miscellaneous	anti-depressant		Roerig	Tablet (NDC49-5660): 300 mg—light blue—engraved Roerig & 566— bottles of 100 & 1000 **Note:** Primary use is in treatment of manic states and prevention of manic and depressive episodes

Book's Color Code	Brand Name N D C Numbers	Generic/ Chemical Name	Classification	Use	Street Name(s)	Manufacturer	Packaging
	Lithium Carbonate 54-2527	lithium carbonate	miscellaneous	anti-depressant		Philips Roxane Labs	Capsule (NDC54-2527): 300 mg—flesh colored—bottles of 100 & 1000 **Note:** Primary use is in treatment of manic states and prevention of manic and depressive episodes
	Lithonate 32-7512	lithium carbonate	miscellaneous	anti-depressant		Rowell	Capsule (NDC32-7512): 300 mg—flesh colored—imprinted Rowell— bottles of 100 & 1000 **Note:** Primary use is in treatment of manic states and prevention of manic and depressive episodes
	L.S.D.	lysergic acid diethylamide	miscellaneous	halluci-nogenic	Acid, Big D, Sunshine, Cubes, Micro Dots or Brown Dots, Barrels, Purple Haze, The Ticket, The Animal, The Beast, The Chief, Crackers, The Hawk, Lucy in the Sky with Diamonds, Trips, Twenty-five	Sandoz (for research)	Mostly private and illegal
	Luminal 24-OX76 24-OX77	phenobarbital	barbiturate	sedative & anti-spasmodic	Downers, Phennies, Purple Hearts, Barbs, Goofballs	Winthrop	Tablets: 16 mg (1/4 gr) (NDC24-OX76) 32 mg (1/2 gr) (NDC24-OX77) Both sugarcoated—oval—bottles of 100 Solutions: For injection—Ampules—130 mg (2 gr)/1 ml—boxes of 100 Vials—10 ml—150 mg (2½ gr)/ml—boxes of 1

	Drug	Generic	Class	Type	Street Names	Manufacturer	Description
	Marijuana **Illegal**	cannabis sativa	miscellaneous	halluci-nogenic	Grass, Pot, Cannabis, Joint, Mary Jane, Tea, Hemp, Bhang, Charas, Ganja, Gage, Gungeon, (Acapulco, Panama, or other) Gold, Panama Red, Weed, Boo, Lid, OJ (opium joint), Mexican Green, Brown Weed, Locoweed, Rainy-Day Woman, Hay, Herb, Wheat, Belyando Sprue	**Illegal**	**Illegal** **Note:** Smoked or taken orally
	Marplan 4-0032	isocarboxazid	monoamine oxidase inhibitor	anti-depressant		Roche	Tablets (NDC4-0032): 10 mg—peach colored—uncoated—imprinted ROCHE—bottles of 100 & 1000
	Mebaral 24-OM31 24-OM32 24-OM33 24-OM34	mephobarbital	barbiturate	sedative & anxiolytic	Barbs, Downers, Goofballs	Winthrop	White tablets: 32 mg (1/2 gr) (NDC24-OM31)—small, scored—2 dots on top, 1 dot on bottom—bottles of 250 & 1000 50 mg (3/4 gr) (NDC24-OM32)—imprinted with 4 lines, 1/2 length of tab, to form open square 100 mg (1½ gr) (NDC24-OM33)—large dot in center 200 mg (3 gr) (NDC24-OM34)—largest of 4—scored—2 dots on top, 1 dot on bottom Last three dosages (50, 100, 200 mg) supplied in bottles of 250 All tablets have W on reverse side

Book's Color Code	Brand Name N D C Numbers	Generic/ Chemical Name	Classification	Use	Street Name(s)	Manufacturer	Packaging
	Medigesic 184-0306	mephenesin, salicylamide	antianxiety	analgesic		Medics Phar. Corp.	Tablets (NDC184-0306): 300 mg mephenesin & 300 mg salicylamide—bottles of 100 & 1000
	Medomin	hepta-barbital	barbiturate	hypnotic & sedative	Barbs, Downers, Goofballs	Geigy	Tablets: 200 mg—white, double-scored—bottles of 50 **Note:** Product discontinued, but quantities of the tablets still may be in circulation
	Mellaril 78-0002 78-0003 78-0004 78-0005 78-0006 78-0007 78-0001	thioridazine	phenothiazine	major tranquilizer		Sandoz	Tablets: 10 mg (NDC78-0002)—bright chartreuse 25 mg (NDC78-0003)—light tan 50 mg (NDC78-0004)—white 100 mg (NDC78-0005)—light chartreuse 150 mg (NDC78-0006)—yellow 200 mg (NDC78-0007)—pink All tablets coated, imprinted SANDOZ on one side, dosage on other All tablets come in bottles of 100 & 1000 Concentrate (NDC78-0001): 30 mg/ml—light yellow, syrupy base—bitter tasting—odorless—bottles of 4 fl oz and 1 pint
	Meper-idine	meperidine HCl	narcotic	narcotic, analgesic			Produced by 10 manufacturers under generic name as sterile solutions for SC, IM, IV injections These manufacturers also produce tablets as follows: Blue Line: 50 mg—bottles of 100 & 1000 Lannett: 50 mg—bottles of 100, 500, 1000 Premo: 50 mg—bottles of 100, 250, 1000 100 mg—bottles of 100, 500, 1000 Wyeth: 50 mg—Redipak box of 25s **Note:** See **Demerol**

Mepro-bamate	meprobamate	antianxiety	sedative & anxiolytic	Downers	Many (33)	Under its generic name and in dosages of 200 & 400 mg, 33 manufacturers produce this drug. **Note:** Same as **Meprospan, Equanil, Kesso-Bamate, Meprotabs, Miltown,** and others Overdosage may cause chills, fever, peripheral edema, possibly convulsions, vasomotor and respiratory collapse, coma, shock, and cardiac arrest
Mepro-span 37-1401 37-1301	meprobamate	antianxiety	sedative & anxiolytic	Downers	Wallace	Capsules: 200 mg (NDC37-1401)—yellow & clear—WALLACE and code number imprinted in red on clear half, 200 on other half 400 mg (NDC37-1301)—blue & clear—WALLACE and code imprinted in red on clear half, 400 on other half **Note:** See **Meprobamate**
Meprotabs 37-1501	meprobamate	antianxiety	sedative & anxiolytic	Downers	Wallace	Tablets (NDC37-1501): 400 mg—white coated—imprinted Wallace 37-1501 in red **Note:** See **Meprobamate**
Meprotil 474-4000	meprobamate	antianxiety	sedative & anxiolytic	Downers	Bruner Tillman Co.	Tablets (NDC474-4000): 400 mg—bottles of 100, 1000 **Note:** See **Meprobamate**
Mescaline Illegal	from Peyote cactus (Lophophora Williamsi)	miscellaneous	halluci-nogenic	Buttons, Mesc, Peyote, Cactus, Topi, The Bad Seed	**Illegal**	**Illegal**
Meth-adone 29-2860 9-0509	methadone HCl	narcotic	narcotic analgesic; CNS depressant; used in treatment of morphine and heroin addiction	Dolls, Dollies	Semed—NDC29-2860 Upjohn—NDC9-0509	Both manufacturers make sterile solutions (10 mg/ml) in 10 ml and 30 ml vials for SC and IM use **Note:** Antidote: **Nalline** (5-10 mg IM or IV)

Book's Color Code	Brand Name N D C Numbers	Generic/ Chemical Name	Classification	Use	Street Name(s)	Manufacturer	Packaging
	Meth- amphet- amine HCl	methamphet- amine HCl	amphetamine	stimulant	Crystal, Speed, Meth, Bombitas, Uppers		Following manufacturers supply this drug under its generic name: American Quinine: Tablets, oral (NDC517-0842)—5 mg—bottles of 1000 Robinson: Parenteral solution—20 mg/cc, in 30 cc vials Tablets—5 mg—bottles of 100 & 1000 Truxton, C.O.: Tablets—5 mg—bottles of 1000
	Meth- edrine	methamphet- amine HCl	amphetamine	stimulant	Crystal, Speed, Meth, Bombitas or Bombidas, Cartwheels, Coast to Coasts, Crank, Crossroads, Uppers	Burroughs Wellcome	(See METHAMPHETAMINE) Elixir: 66 mg/cc Sterile solution: 20 mg/cc **Note:** Same as **Desoxyn, Desoxyephedrine, Norodin, Desyphed, Syndrox** (McNeil, NDC45-0409)
	Miltown 37-1101 37-1001 37-1201	meprobamate	antianxiety	sedative & anxiolytic	Downers	Wallace	Tablets: 200 mg (NDC37-1101)—white—coated—imprinted Wallace 37-1101 400 mg (NDC37-1001)—white—scored W— imprinted Wallace 37-1001 Sterile solution (NDC37-1201): IM 400 mg/5 cc **Note:** See **Meprobamate**
	Morphine There are 37 NDCs	opium alkaloid	narcotic	narcotic, analgesic	Morf or Morph, M, White Stuff, Dreamer	Various phar- maceutical houses (12)	Tablets: oral—5 mg, 8 mg, 10 mg, 15 mg Tablets: for hypodermic use Sterile solutions for parenteral use **Note:** Antidote: **Nalline** (5-10 mg IM or IV)

Name / NDC	Generic	Class	Use	Slang	Manufacturer	Description
Nardil 47-0270	phenelzine sulfate	monoamine oxidase inhibitor	anti-depressant		Warner-Chilcott	Tablets (NDC47-0270): 15 mg—pale red—coated—black W/C imprint—bottles of 100
Navane 49-5710 49-5720 49-5730 49-5740 49-5750 49-5760	thiothixene	pheno-thiazine	sedative & anxiolytic		Roerig	Capsules: 1 mg (NDC49-5710)—yellow & orange—black "1 mg" imprinted on each half / 2 mg (NDC49-5720)—yellow & blue—black "2 mg" imprinted on each half / 5 mg (NDC49-5730)—white & orange—black "5 mg" imprinted on each half / 10 mg (NDC49-5740)—white & blue—black "10 mg" imprinted on each half / All strengths come in bottles of 100 & 1000 / Concentrate (NDC49-5750): 5 mg/cc—colorless—aromatic—pleasant-tasting—supplied in 4 oz dropper bottles / Solution (NDC49-5760): intramuscular—2 mg/cc—packages of 10 vials
Nebralin 43-0028	pentobarbital and mephenesin	barbiturate	sedative & anxiolytic	Phennies, Barbs, Downers	Dorsey	Tablets (NDC43-0028): oblong—light blue—90 mg pentobarbital & 425 mg mephenesin—engraved DORSEY—bottles of 50

Book's Color Code	Brand Name N D C Numbers	Generic/ Chemical Name	Classification	Use	Street Name(s)	Manufacturer	Packaging
	Nembutal Sodium 74-3120 74-3150 74-3114 74-6870 74-3142 74-3272 74-3148 74-3145 74-3164 74-3778	sodium pentobarbital	barbiturate	sedative	Yellow Jackets, Nimbys, Nemmies, Nebbies, Barbs, Downers, Menish	Abbott	Capsules: 30 mg (NDC74-3120)—yellow—" ⊐ " imprint—bottles of 100 & 1000 50 mg (NDC74-3150)—clear with yellow cap (since 1972, clear with red cap)—" ⊐ " on one half and ABBOTT imprinted on other half—bottles of 100, 500, 1000 100 mg (NDC74-3114)—yellow—" ⊐ " on one half and ABBOTT imprinted on other half—bottles of 100, 500, 1000 All also in strip packages of 25 & Abbo-Pac-Unit-of-use packages of 100 Nembutal Gradumet (NDC74-6870): 100 mg—blue tablet—bottles of 100 Nembutal Elixir (NDC74-3142): 20 mg/teaspoon—bottles of 1 pt & 1 gallon Suppositories: 30 mg (NDC74-3272), 60 mg (NDC74-3148), 120 mg (NDC74-3145), 200 mg (NDC74-3164) All in boxes of 12 & 100 Solutions (injectable): 100 mg (1½ gr)—2 ml ampules 250 mg (4 gr)—5 ml ampules 50 mg/ml—20 & 50 ml multiple dose vials (NDC74-3778)
	Niamid	nialamide	monoamine oxidase inhibitor	anti-depressant		Pfizer	Tablets: 25 mg—pink 100 mg—orange Both scored—Pfizer monogram—in bottles of 100 **Note:** Product has been discontinued, but quantities still may be in circulation

Name / NDC	Generic	Class	Action	Street names	Manufacturer	Description
Noctec 3-0623 3-0626 3-0627	chloral hydrate	barbiturate-like	sedative & hypnotic	Knock-out Drops, Mickey Finn (with alcohol), Joy Juice	Squibb	Capsules: 250 mg (3¾ gr) (NDC3-0623)—bottles of 100 500 mg (7½ gr) (NDC3-0626)—bottles of 100 & Unimatic Single Dose Packs of 100 Both capsules red, imprinted with Squibb & appropriate NDC number in white Syrup (NDC3-0627): Orange flavored—500 mg/5 ml—rose colored—fruity odor—bottles of 1 pint & 1 gallon **Note:** Patients suffer gastric distress Quick circulatory collapse may occur
Noludar 4-0019 4-0016 4-0017	methyprylon	barbiturate-like	sedative & anxiolytic	Downers, Goofballs	Roche	Capsules: 300 mg (NDC4-0019)—amethyst & white—black ROCHE 19 imprint—bottles of 100 & 500 Tablets: 50 mg (NDC4-0016)—scored—monogrammed HLR—bottles of 100 200 mg (NDC4-0017)—scored—monogrammed R—bottles of 100 & 500 **Note:** Do not provoke vomiting; it could result in sudden cessation of respirations Patients suffering from large overdose may have to be intubated as a precautionary measure
Norpramin 73-4800 73-4801	desipramine HCl	tricyclic	anti-depressant		Lakeside	Tablets: 25 mg (NDC73-4800)—yellow—bottles of 50, 500, 1000—imprinted 11 50 mg (NDC73-4801)—light green—bottles of 50, 250, 1000—imprinted 12 Both round—coated—imprinted with LAKESIDE trademark in black

Book's Color Code	Brand Name N D C Numbers	Generic/ Chemical Name	Classification	Use	Street Name(s)	Manufacturer	Packaging

	Opium 2-OY77 274-2818 (camphorated) 527-0766 (camphorated) 8-0330 (w/belladonna)		narcotic	narcotic	Blue Velvet (for Paregoric and Pyribenzamine combination), Big O, Black Stuff, PG (Paregoric), Tar, Op, Hop, Brown Stuff, Black Stuff	Lilly First Texas Pharma- ceuticals Lannett Wyeth	Prepared as straight tincture—oral—10 Gm/100 ml—bottles of 4 oz & 1 pt
							    Very potent
							        Safe dosage is only in drops
							As camphorated opium tincture—oral—pint & gallon bottles
							    Is in wider use primarily for diarrhea
							In suppositories—rectal—as "opium and belladonna"

	Optimil 37-8201 37-8301	methaqualone HCl	barbiturate- like	sedative, hypnotic	Downers, Sopors	Wallace	Capsules: 200 mg (NDC37-8201)—opaque pink cap, clear pink body— imprinted Wallace 37-8201 on cap, 200 on body
							    400 mg (NDC37-8301)—opaque powder blue cap, clear pink body—imprinted Wallace 37-8301 on cap, 400 on body
							Note: Dangerous in combination with alcohol
							    Vomiting, gastric irritation, transient paresthesias or hypotension
							    There may be cutaneous edema, bleeding, pulmonary edema, hepatic damage or renal insufficiency

	Pagitane 2-OC16 2-OC17	cycrimine HCl	antiParkinson	antiParkinson		Lilly	Coated tablets: 1.25 mg (NDC2-OC16)—orange
							    2.5 mg (NDC2-OC17)—brown
							        Bottles of 100 & 1000

	Pantopon 4-1918	hydrochlorides of opium alkaloids	narcotic	narcotic, sedative, hypnotic	Downers	Roche	Ampules (NDC4-1918): 20 mg (1/3 gr)/1 ml—boxes of 10 ampules for IM & SC use **Note:** Antidote: Use **Lorfan**

	Name	Generic	Class	Action	Slang	Manufacturer	Description
	Parest 71-0572 71-0574	methaqualone HCl	barbiturate-like	sedative, hypnotic	Downers, Sopors	Parke Davis	Capsules: Parest-200 (NDC71-0572)—light turquoise blue, opaque blue cap & light green opaque body—imprinted PD 572 on each half Parest-400 (NDC71-0574)—standard blue cap & light green opaque body—imprinted PD 574 on each half Both capsule strengths are supplied in bottles of 100 & unit dose packages of 100 (10 strips of 10 capsules each)
	Parnate 7-ON71	tranyl-cypromine	monoamine oxidase inhibitor	anti-depressant		Smith, Kline & French	Tablet (NDC7-ON71): 10 mg—red—coated—black SKF N71 imprint—bottles of 100 & 1000
	Parsidol 47-0320 47-0321 47-0322	ethopropazine HCl	pheno-thiazine	antiParkinson		Warner-Chilcott	Tablets: oral—10 mg (NDC47-0320), 50 mg (NDC47-0321), 100 mg (NDC47-0322)—bottles of 100, engraved W/C
	Pentothal 74-3158 74-3159 74-6181 74-3314 74-6423 74-3329 74-6431 74-6121 74-6435 74-6128 74-6672 74-6175 74-7236	sodium thiopental	barbiturate	sedative & hypnotic	Downers, Barbs, Goofballs	Abbott	In various strengths for injection and as a rectal suspension

Book's Color Code	Brand Name N D C Numbers	Generic/ Chemical Name	Classification	Use	Street Name(s)	Manufacturer	Packaging
	Permitil 85-OWKJ 85-OWBK 85-OWGB 85-OWDR 85-OWFF 85-OWFG 85-OWJP	fluphenazine HCl	pheno- thiazine	major tranquilizer		Schering	Tablets: Chronotabs (NDC85-OWKJ)—1 mg—coated—yellow— bottles of 60, 250, 1000 0.25 mg (NDC85-OWBK)—coated—green—bottles of 50 & 500 1.0 mg (NDC85-OWGB)—yellow—bottles of 1000 2.5 mg (NDC85-OWDR)—peach—bottles of 50 & 1000 5.0 mg (NDC85-OWFF)—pink—bottles of 50 & 1000 10.0 mg (NDC85-OWFG)—reddish—bottles of 1000 All except 0.25 mg & 1mg are uncoated—scored—engraved W/L Oral concentrate (NDC85-OWJP): 5 mg/ml—colorless—odorless— tasteless—bottles of 120 ml
	Pertofrane 75-3511 75-3521	desipramine HCl	tricyclic	anti- depressant		USV Phar- maceutical	Capsules: 25 mg (NDC75-3511)—pink—bottles of 100, 1000 50 mg (NDC75-3521)—maroon & pink—bottles of 100 Both have USV imprint on body and cap
	Phenergan 8-0019 8-0027 8-0227 8-0161 8-0212 8-0229 8-0041 8-0228 8-0231	promethazine HCl	pheno- thiazine	anti- histaminic & anxiolytic agent		Wyeth	Tablets: 12.5 mg (NDC8-0019)—grey—scored—bottles of 100 & 1000 & strip pack boxes of 100 25 mg (NDC8-0027)—white—engraved W—vials of 100, bottles of 1000, strip pack boxes of 25 50 mg (NDC8-0227)—pink—vials of 100 Syrup (NDC8-0161): 6.25 mg/teaspoon—pint bottles Syrup Fortis (NDC8-0231): 25 mg/teaspoon—pint bottles Rectal Suppositories: 25 mg (NDC8-0212) & 50 mg (NDC8-0229)— boxes of 12 & 25 Solution: injection—25 mg/ml (NDC8-0041)—IM or IV—packages of 25— 1 ml ampules & 10 ml vials 50 mg/ml (NDC8-0228)—IM only—packages of 25—vials of 10 ml **Note:** This drug comes in combination with **Codeine** for use as an expectorant

Phenoxene 183-0603	chlorphenox- amine HCl	antiParkinson	antiParkinson		Dow Chemical	Tablets (NDC183-0603): oral—50 mg—bottles of 100
Placidyl 74-6649 74-6661 74-6685 74-6630	ethchlorvynol	barbiturate- like	sedative & anxiolytic	Downers	Abbott	Coated tablets: 100 mg—red—no marking 200 mg—red—no marking Capsules: 100 mg (NDC74-6649)—red—bottles of 100 200 mg (NDC74-6661)—red—bottles of 100 500 mg (NDC74-6685)—red—bottles of 100 & 500 750 mg (NDC74-6630)—green—bottles of 100 ABBO-PAC: 100 capsules in strips of 10 capsules each All capsules have ABBOTT imprinted in white
Proketa- zine 8-0251 8-0252 8-0253 8-0274	carphenazine maleate	pheno- thiazine	major tranquilizer		Wyeth	Tablets: 12.5 mg (NDC8-0251)—yellow 25 mg (NDC8-0252)—peach 50 mg (NDC8-0253)—pink All are coated—round—in vials of 50 & bottles of 500 Concentrate (NDC8-0274): Syrup—50 mg/cc
Prolixin 3-0863 3-0864 3-0877 3-0820 3-0586 3-0824	fluphenazine HCl	pheno- thiazine	major tranquilizer		Squibb	Tablets: 1 mg (NDC3-0863)—round—pink—coated—no marking—bottles of 50 & 100 2.5 mg (NDC3-0864)—round—yellow—coated—no marking—bottles of 50, 100, 500 5.0 mg (NDC3-0877)—round—green—coated—Squibb trademark imprinted—bottles of 50 & 500 Prolixin Elixir (NDC3-0820): 0.5 mg/ml—orange flavor, color & odor—bottles of 60 ml & 1 pint Solution (NDC3-0586): injection—10 cc multiple dose vials—2.5 mg/cc Prolixin Enanthate (NDC3-0824): 25 mg/1cc—vials of 5 cc—Unimatic single dose—preassembled syringes of 1 cc—cartridge units of 1 cc

Book's Color Code	Brand Name NDC Numbers	Generic/ Chemical Name	Classification	Use	Street Name(s)	Manufacturer	Packaging
	Quaalude 67-0712 67-0714	methaqualone	barbiturate-like	sedative, hypnotic	Sopors, Qs, Luds, "The Love Drug," Quads	W. H. Rorer	Uncoated tablets: 150 mg (NDC67-0712)—engraved RORER 712 300 mg (NDC67-0714)—engraved RORER 714 Both are white—scored—in bottles of 100, 500, 1000 **Note:** Overdosage also causes vomiting, gastric irritation, transient paresthesias, hypotension (because of direct action on heart), possibly pulmonary edema Dangerous in combination with alcohol
	Quide 183-0052 183-0053	piperacetazine	pheno-thiazine	major tranquilizer		Dow Chemical	Tablets: 10 mg (NDC183-0052)—orange 25 mg (NDC183-0053)—yellow Both are film coated, in bottles of 100 & 1000
	Repoise 31-6805 31-6810 31-6825	butaperazine	pheno-thiazine	major tranquilizer		A. H. Robins	Tablets: 5 mg (NDC31-6805)—yellow 10 mg (NDC31-6810)—green 25 mg (NDC31-6825)—orange All are film coated—engraved AHR—in bottles of 100 & 500
	Ritalin 83-0007 83-0003 83-0034 83-7432	methyl-phenidate HCl	miscellaneous	stimulant	Uppers	CIBA	Uncoated tablets: 5 mg (NDC83-0007)—pale yellow—bottles of 100, 500, 1000 10 mg (NDC83-0003)—pale green—bottles of 100, 500, 1000 & strip dispensers of 100 20 mg (NDC83-0034)—peach—bottles of 100 & 1000 All engraved CIBA, all scored (For the military services): 10 mg—bottles of 1000—Stock #6505-584-3179 (For the VA): 10 mg—bottles of 1000—Stock #6505-584-3179A 20 mg—bottles of 1000—Stock #6505-584-3181A Solution: multiple dose vials—100 mg/10 ml Injection (NDC83-7432): sterile powder—100 mg/10 ml for IV, IM, SC

	Drug	Generic	Class	Type	Street Names	Manufacturer	Dosage Forms
	Robaxin 31-7429 31-7449 31-7409	meth-ocarbamol	antianxiety	sedative & anxiolytic	Downers	A. H. Robins	Tablets: 500 mg (NDC31-7429)—compressed 750 mg (NDC31-7449)—capsule-shaped Both scored—white—engraved AHR—in bottles of 50 & 500 Solution (NDC31-7409): sterile & intravenous—100 mg/ml—intramuscular— 10 ml ampules in boxes of 5 & 25

	**Seconal,
	Seconal
	Sodium**
	2-OA24
	2-OF72
	2-OF42
	2-OF40
	2-0517
	2-0514
	2-0505
	2-0511
	2-OX83
	2-OP68
	2-ON32
	2-ON72
	2-OX44
		secobarbital,
		sodium
		secobarbital
			barbiturate	sedative	Reds, Seggy,
					Red Devils,
					Mexican Reds,
					Pinks, Red Birds,
					Red Lillies,
					Phenos, Downers
						Lilly	Enseals (NDC2-OA24): Seconal sodium 100 mg (1½ gr)—bottles of 100
							Capsules: Seconal
							    30 mg (1/2 gr) (NDC2-OF72)—orange—imprinted Lilly F72 in white—
							        packages of 100 & 500
							    50 mg (3/4 gr) (NDC2-OF42)—orange—imprinted Lilly F42 in white—
							        packages of 100, 500, 5000
							        Both in 10 strips of 10 individually labeled blisters
							    100 mg (1½ gr) (NDC2-OF40)—orange—imprinted Lilly F40—
							        packages of 100, 500, 5000
							        Also in 10 strips of 10 individually labeled blisters
							        Strip packages of individually sealed capsules
							Suppositories: 30 mg (1/2 gr) (NDC2-0517)
							        60 mg (1 gr) (NDC2-0514)
							        120 mg (2 gr) (NDC2-0505)
							        200 mg (3 gr) (NDC2-0511)
							        All in packages of 12
							Powder (NDC2-OX83): oral bulk—in 1/2 oz bottle
							Ampules (NDC2-OP68): 250 mg/ampule
							Injection (NDC2-ON32): sterile sol.—50 mg/ml
							Injection (NDC2-ON72): sterile sol.—hyporet 100 mg/2 cc
							Seconal Elixir (NDC2-OX44): 22 mg/5 cc

Book's Color Code	Brand Name N D C Numbers	Generic/ Chemical Name	Classification	Use	Street Name(s)	Manufacturer	Packaging
	Serax 8-0317 8-0051 8-0006 8-0052	oxazepam	antianxiety	sedative & anxiolytic	Downers	Wyeth	Uncoated tablets (NDC8-0317): 15 mg—yellow—Wyeth monogram impressed—vials of 100 Capsules: 10 mg (NDC8-0051)—white body, pink cap 15 mg (NDC8-0006)—white body, red cap 30 mg (NDC8-0052)—white body, maroon cap Each capsule half imprinted Wyeth and dosage strength All strengths in bottles of 100 & 500 Redipak (Strip Pack) in boxes of 25
	Serentil 78-0011 78-0012 78-0013 78-0014 78-0010	mesoridazine besylate	pheno-thiazine	major tranquilizer		Sandoz	Tablets: 10 mg (NDC78-0011), 25 mg (NDC78-0012), 50 mg (NDC78-0013), 100 mg (NDC78-0014) All dark red—imprinted Sandoz & dosage—bottles of 100 Solution (NDC78-0010): ampules—25 mg/1 ml—for parenteral use
	Sinequan 69-5340 69-5350 69-0536	doxepin HCl	Treat as tricyclic	anti-depressant & antianxiety		Pfizer	Capsules: 10 mg (NDC69-5340)—pink body, red cap—imprinted Pfizer 534—bottles of 100 25 mg (NDC69-5350)—pink body, blue cap—imprinted Pfizer 535—bottles of 100 & 1000 50 mg (NDC69-0536)—pink and rose—imprinted Pfizer 536—bottles of 100 & 1000
	Solacen 37-7001 37-7101	tybamate	antianxiety	sedative & anxiolytic	Downers	Wallace	Capsules: 250 mg (NDC37-7001)—yellow—sealed oval 350 mg (NDC37-7101)—yellow—sealed capsule Both in bottles of 100

	Name	Generic	Classification	Action	Slang	Manufacturer	Supplied
	Somnafac, Somnafac Fourte 58-1900 58-1901	methaqualone HCl	barbiturate-like	sedative, hypnotic	Luds, Sopors, Qs, "The Love Drug," Quads	Smith, Miller & Patch	Capsules: Somnafac capsule (NDC58-1900)—two-tone blue—oral—200 mg—bottles of 100 Somnafac Fourte capsule (NDC58-1901)—400 mg—dark blue—bottles of 30 & 100 **Notes:** Overdosage with **Somnafac Fourte** may cause cutaneous edema, bleeding, pulmonary edema and hypotension because of direct action on heart Overdosage with **Somnafac** may also cause vomiting, gastric irritation and transient paresthesias Dangerous in combination with alcohol
	Sopor 94-0084 94-0085 94-0086	methaqualone	barbiturate-like	sedative, hypnotic	Qs, Sopors, Luds, "The Love Drug," Quads	Arnar-Stone	Uncoated tablets: 75 mg (NDC94-0084)—green—bottles of 100 & 500 150 mg (NDC94-0085)—white—bottles of 100, 500, 1000 300 mg (NDC94-0086)—pink—bottles of 100, 500, 1000 All tablets engraved AS **Note:** See **Somnafac**
	Sparine 8-0202 8-0029 8-0028 8-0200 8-0201 8-0203 8-0210 8-0238	promazine HCl	pheno-thiazine	major tranquilizer		Wyeth	Coated tablets: 10 mg (NDC8-0202)—green 25 mg (NDC8-0029)—yellow 50 mg (NDC8-0028)—orange 100 mg (NDC8-0200)—pink 200 mg (NDC8-0201)—red All in vials of 50 & bottles of 500 Syrup (NDC8-0203): 10 mg/5 ml—bottles of 4 fluid ounces Concentrate: Liquid (NDC8-0210): 30 mg/ml—bottles of 4 fluid ounces Syrup (NDC8-0238): 100 mg/ml—bottles of 30 fluid ounces Solutions: sterile—IM 50 mg/ml—vials of 2 ml & 10 ml sterile—IM, IV—25 mg/ml—vials of 10 ml 50 mg/ml, 25 mg/ml also supplied in unit-tubex of 10—1 ml, 10—2 ml

Book's Color Code	Brand Name N D C Numbers	Generic/ Chemical Name	Classification	Use	Street Name(s)	Manufacturer	Packaging
	Stelazine 484-0503 484-0504 484-0506 484-0507 484-0501 484-0502	trifluo- perazine HCl	pheno- thiazine	major tranquilizer		Smith, Kline & French	Tablets: blue—coated—dosages of 1 mg (NDC484-0503), 2 mg (NDC484-0504), 5 mg (NDC484-0506), 10 mg (NDC484-0507)— SKF monogram, dosage imprinted on each—bottles of 100 & 1000 Concentrate (NDC484-0501): bitter taste—vanilla odor—10 mg/ml— 2 fl oz bottles—cartons of 12 bottles Solutions (NDC484-0502): sterile—IM, IV—2 mg/ml—10 cc vials— multiple dose vials—10 mg/ml—boxes of 1 & 20
	Stental Extentabs 31-9449	pheno- barbital	barbiturate	sedative	Downers	A. H. Robins	Tablets (NDC31-9449): 48.6 mg—light pink—coated—monogrammed AHR in black—bottles of 100 & 500
	Suavitil 6-0024	benactyzine HCl	antianxiety	anxiolytic	Downers	Merck Sharp & Dohme	Tablets (NDC6-0024): oral—1 mg—bottles of 100
	Suvren 46-0732 46-0733	captodiamine	antihistamine	sedative & anxiolytic	Downers	Ayerst	Tablets: 50 mg (NDC46-0732)—red 100 mg (NDC46-0733)—peach Both in bottles of 100
	Talwin 24-OT21 24-OT11 24-OT12 24-OT13 24-OT16	pentazocine as hydro- chloride	narcotic	analgesic		Winthrop	Tablets (NDC24-OT21): 50 mg—peach color—engraved WINTHROP— bottles of 100 Solutions: (pentazocine as lactate) for parenteral use—IM, SC, IV— sterile—ampules 30 mg/ml (NDC24-OT11) 45 mg/1½ ml (NDC24-OT12) 60 mg/2 ml (NDC24-OT13) 30 mg/ml in 10 ml vials (NDC24-OT16) **Note:** For respiratory depression caused by overdosage of **Talwin, Narcan** (naloxone) is the specific and effective antagonist. If **Narcan** is not

available, use **Ritalin** (methylphenidate)
Nalorphine and levallorphan are NOT effective against respiratory
depression caused by overdosage with this drug

Taractan
4-0045
4-0046
4-0047
4-0049
4-1010
4-1926
	chlor-
	prothixene
		pheno-
		thiazine
			sedative &
			anxiolytic
					Roche	Tablets: 10 mg (NDC4-0045)—light coral 25 mg (NDC4-0046)—light coral
						    50 mg (NDC4-0047)—dark coral 100 mg (NDC4-0049)—dark coral
						All are round—coated—in graduated sizes—with appropriate NDC
						    imprinted in black—bottles of 100 & 500
						Concentrate (NDC4-1010): 100 mg/5 ml (teaspoon)—fruit flavored—
						    1 pint bottles
						Ampules (NDC4-1926): 25 mg/2 ml—boxes of 10

Thorazine
7-OT73
7-OT74
7-OT76
7-OT77
7-OT79
7-OT63
7-OT64
7-OT66
7-OT67
7-OT69
7-OT72
7-OT47
7-OT49
7-OT60
7-OT61
7-OT70
7-OT71
	chlor-
	promazine
		pheno-
		thiazine
			major
			tranquilizer
					Smith, Kline
					& French
						Tablets: 10 mg (NDC7-OT73), 25 mg (NDC7-OT74), 50 mg (NDC7-OT76),
						    100 mg (NDC7-OT77), 200 mg (NDC7-OT79)—dark orange—coated—
						    imprinted SKF and dosage—bottles of 100 and 1000
						Spansules: 30 mg/one dot (NDC7-OT63) 75 mg/two dots (NDC7-OT64)
						    150 mg/three dots (NDC7-OT66) 200 mg/four dots (NDC7-OT67)
						    300 mg/five dots and bars (NDC7-OT69)
						    All are sustained release capsules. Transparent half reveals multicolored
						    granules. Orange half has SKF monogram and white dots according to
						    dosage as above. All in bottles of 50 & 500, except 300 mg which comes in
						    bottles of 50
						Syrup (NDC7-OT72): 10 mg/5 ml—in 4 fl oz bottles
						Concentrate: light straw color—odorless—bitter tasting—30 mg/ml—
						    120 ml bottles, cartons of 36 bottles—also in 1 gal bottles (NDC7-OT47)
						    100 mg/ml—in 9 fl oz bottles (NDC7-OT49)
						Ampules: 1 ml (NDC7-OT60), 2 ml (NDC7-OT61), 25 mg/ml—
						    boxes of 6, 100 & 500
						Multiple dose 10 ml vials—25 mg/ml—boxes of 1, 20, 100
						Suppositories: 25 mg (NDC7-OT70) & 100 mg (NDC7-OT71)—both carry
						    orange stripes with black dosage imprint—boxes of 6

Book's Color Code	Brand Name N D C Numbers	Generic/ Chemical Name	Classification	Use	Street Name(s)	Manufacturer	Packaging
	Tindal 85-OBBA	acetophen- azine maleate	pheno- thiazine	major tranquilizer		Schering	Tablets (NDC85-OBBA): 20 mg—coated—peach colored—red Schering trademarks imprinted—bottles of 100 & 1000
	Tofranil 28-0021 28-0011 28-0074 28-0065	imipramine HCl	tricyclic	anti- depressant		Geigy	Tablets: 10 mg (NDC28-0021)—triangular—coated—coral colored—black GEIGY imprint—bottles of 100 & 1000 25 mg (NDC28-0011)—round—coated—coral colored—black GEIGY imprint—bottles of 100, 1000, 5000—also unit strip packages of 100 & 1000 50 mg (NDC28-0074)—round—coated—coral colored—white GEIGY imprint—bottles of 100, 1000, 5000—also unit strip packages of 100 & 1000 Solution (NDC28-0065): Ampules—IM—25 mg/2 ml—boxes of 10 & 50
	Trancopal 24-OT73 24-OT74	chlor- mezanone	antianxiety	sedative & anxiolytic	Downers	Winthrop	Uncoated tablets (Caplets): 100 mg (NDC24-OT73)—peach—bottles of 100 200 mg (NDC24-OT74)—green—bottles of 100 & 1000 Both scored W—capsule shaped
	Triavil 6-0914 6-0921 6-0934 6-0946	perphenazine & amitriptyline HCl	phenothiazine & tricyclic	tranquilizer— anti- depressant		Merck Sharp & Dohme	Tablets: blue (NDC6-0914)—2 mg perphenazine & 10 mg amitriptyline HCl orange (NDC6-0921)—2 mg perphenazine & 25 mg amitriptyline HCl salmon (NDC6-0934)—4 mg perphenazine & 10 mg amitriptyline HCl yellow (NDC6-0946)—4 mg perphenazine & 25 mg amitriptyline HCl All triangular—film coated—imprinted MSD—bottles of 50, 500— also single unit packages of 100

	Generic	Class	Use	Street names	Manufacturer	Forms
Trilafon 85-OADH 85-OADK 85-OADJ 85-OADM 85-OADX 85-OADT 85-OADS 85-OAEC	perphenazine	phenothiazine	major tranquilizer		Schering	Tablets: 2 mg (NDC85-OADH)—black Schering imprint 5 mg (NDC85-OADK)—blue Schering & ADK imprint 8 mg (NDC85-OADJ)—green Schering imprint 16 mg (NDC85-OADM)—red Schering & ADM imprint All are white—coated—in bottles of 50 & 500 Repetabs (NDC85-OADX): 8 mg—bottles of 30, 100, 1000 Concentrate (NDC85-OADT): raspberry flavor & odor—colorless—16 mg/5 ml—4 oz bottles Syrup (NDC85-OADS): 2 mg/5 ml—4 oz bottles Injections (NDC85-OAEC): ampules—5 mg/ml—IM, IV—boxes of 6 & 100 10 ml multidose vials
Tuinal 2-OF64 2-OF65 2-OF66	sodium amobarbital & sodium secobarbital	barbiturates in combination	sedative & hypnotic	Rainbows, Double Troubles, Tooies, Red and Blues	Lilly	Capsules: 50 mg (3/4 gr) (NDC2-OF64)—bottles of 100 & 1000 100 mg (1½ gr) (NDC2-OF65)—bottles of 100, 1000, 5000; in 10 strips of 10 individually labeled blisters, each with 1 capsule 200 mg (3 gr) (NDC2-OF66)—bottles of 100, 1000, 5000; strip packages of individually sealed capsules; 10 strips of 10 individually labeled blisters, each with 1 capsule All: blue body, orange cap—LILLY & NDC imprinted on body
Tybatran 31-9715 31-9750 31-9765	tybamate	antianxiety	sedative & anxiolytic	Downers	A. H. Robins	Capsules: 125 mg (NDC31-9715)—AHR 125 white imprint 250 mg (NDC31-9750)—AHR 250 white imprint 350 mg (NDC31-9765)—AHR 350 white imprint All are sealed—soft gelatine—green—in bottles of 100 & 500

Book's Color Code	Brand Name N D C Numbers	Generic/ Chemical Name	Classification	Use	Street Name(s)	Manufacturer	Packaging
	Ultran 2-OT97 2-QH01	phena-glycodol	antianxiety	sedative & anxiolytic	Downers	Lilly	Tablets (NDC2-OT97): 200 mg—capsule shaped—scored Capsules (NDC2-OH01): 300 mg—white opaque body, green cap Both in bottles of 100
	Valium 4-0004 4-0005 4-0006 4-1931 4-1932 4-1933	diazepam	antianxiety	sedative & anxiolytic	Downers	Roche	Tablets: 2 mg (NDC4-0004)—white—scored—monogrammed ROCHE 4 5 mg (NDC4-0005)—yellow—scored—monogrammed ROCHE 5 10 mg (NDC4-0006)—blue—scored—monogrammed ROCHE 6 All are uncoated, supplied in bottles of 100 & 500; also in Tel-E-Dose packages of 1000 Solutions: (ampules)—5 mg/ml 2 ml (NDC4-1931)—boxes of 10 10 ml (NDC4-1932)—boxes of 1 2 ml—boxes of 10 Tel-E-Ject disposable syringes (NDC4-1933)
	Valmid 2-OJ12	ethinamate	barbiturate-like	sedative & anxiolytic	Downers	Lilly	Tablet (NDC2-OJ12): 0.5 Gm—peach colored—scored Lilly J12— bottles of 100
	Vesprin 3-0921 3-0922 3-0923 3-0935 3-0987 3-0920	triflu-promazine HCl	phenothiazine	major tranquilizer		Squibb	Tablets: 10 mg (NDC3-0921)—pink 25 mg (NDC3-0922)—yellow 50 mg (NDC3-0923)—aqua All are uncoated, have colorless Squibb trademark imprint, are supplied in bottles of 50 & 500 Vesprin High-Potency Suspension (NDC3-0935): 50 mg/5 ml—vanilla flavored—120 ml bottles Vesprin injection—IM, IV—10 mg/ml (NDC3-0987)—multiple dose vials of 10 ml, 20 mg/ml (NDC3-0920), vials of 1 ml

	Generic	Class	Slang/Use	Manufacturer	Description
Vistaril 69-5410 69-5420 69-5430 69-5440	hydroxyzine pamoate	antihistamine	antihistamine Downers & anxiolytic	Pfizer	Capsules: 25 mg (NDC69-5410)—two-tone green—Pfizer imprinted on one half, 541 on other 50 mg (NDC69-5420)—green & white—Pfizer & 542 imprinted on both halves 100 mg (NDC69-5430)—grey & green—Pfizer & 543 imprinted on both halves All above come in bottles of 100 & 500 Oral suspension (NDC69-5440): canary yellow colored—lemon flavor—25 mg/teaspoon—pint bottles Solutions for injections: 25 mg/ml, 50 mg/ml & 100 mg/ml **Notes:** Each packaging of injectable solution has different NDC number, but there are only the above 3 strengths This drug has a minor use as an antiarrhythmic
Vivactil HCl 6-0026 6-0047	protriptyline HCl	tricyclic	anti-depressant	Merck Sharp & Dohme	Tablets: 5 mg (NDC6-0026)—orange 10 mg (NDC6-0047)—yellow Both oval—film coated—supplied in bottles of 100 & 1000 Also in blister strips of 100

Approximate Child and Youth Doses

Expressed as percentage of adult dose

Weight in kilos	Weight in pounds	% of adult dose
4-5	9-11	15%
6-7	12-16	20%
8-9	17-21	25%
10-12	22-27	30%
13-15	28-34	35%
16-18	35-40	40%
19-21	41-46	45%
22-25	47-55	50%
26-29	56-64	55%
30-33	65-74	60%
34-37	75-82	65%
38-41	83-91	70%
42-45	92-99	75%
46-49	100-109	80%
50-54	110-119	85%
55-59	120-130	90%
60-65	131-143	95%

Based on body surface area

Surface area in meters^2 = 0.1 x $\sqrt[3]{\text{weight in kilos}^2}$

Adult surface area figured as 1.65 meters^2

Note: These approximations do not hold for all drugs.

Warning:

Intravenous saline for infants and children should be 0.25% or 0.40% solutions unless otherwise indicated by electrolyte studies. Quantities and rate of flow should be carefully calculated and monitored.

Combined Identification Section

Adipex Ty-Med

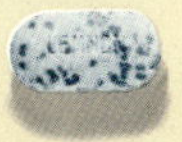

Buticaps

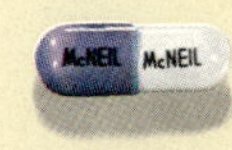 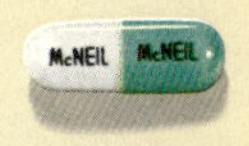

¼ gr.   ½ gr.

Akineton

2 mg.

Butisol Sodium

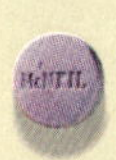 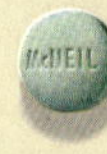 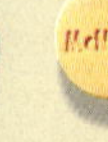 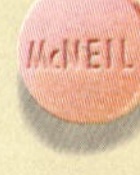

15 mg.   30 mg.   50 mg.   100 mg.

Amytal

 15 mg.   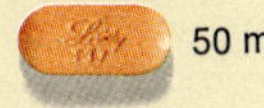 50 mg.

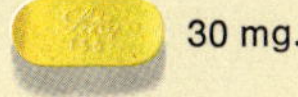 30 mg.   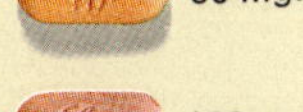 100 mg.

Cogentin

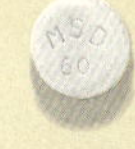 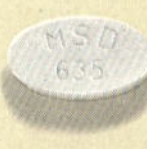 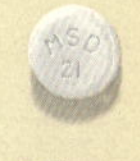

2 mg.   1 mg.   0.5 mg.

Amytal Sodium

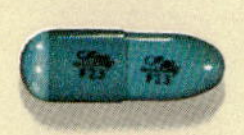 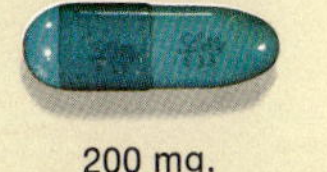

65 mg.   200 mg.

Compazine

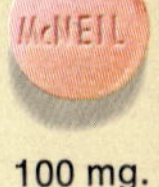

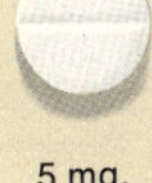 5 mg. (C66)   15 mg. (C46)

10 mg. (C67)   10 mg. (C44)

25 mg. (C69)   30 mg. (C47)

75 mg. (C49)

Artane

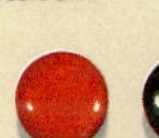 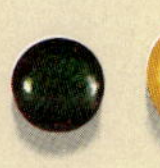 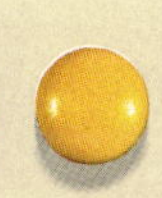

2 mg.   5 mg.   5 mg.

Dartal

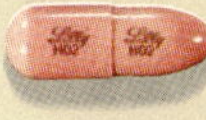 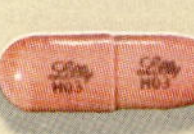

5 mg.   10 mg.

Atarax

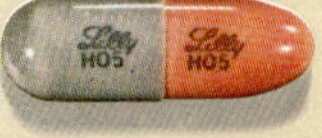 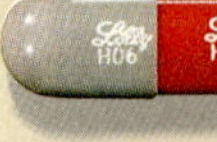 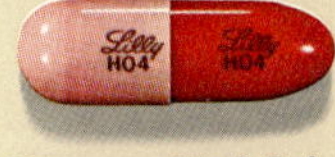 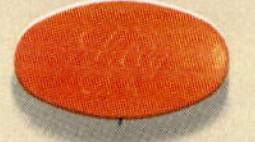

10 mg.   25 mg.   50 mg.   100 mg.

Darvon

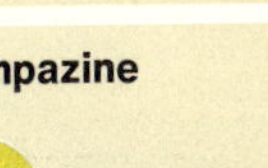 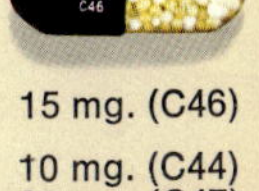

32 mg.   65 mg.

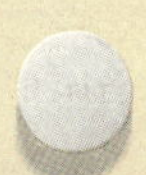

Darvon Compound

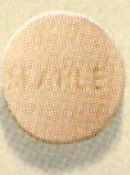

Darvon Compound-65

Darvon with A.S.A.

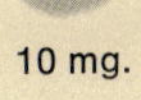

Darvon-N with A.S.A.

Aventyl HCl

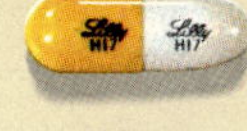 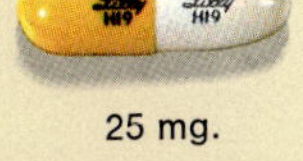

10 mg.   25 mg.

Benadryl

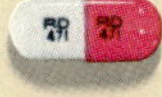 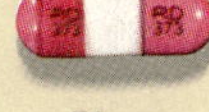

25 mg.   50 mg.

Benzedrine

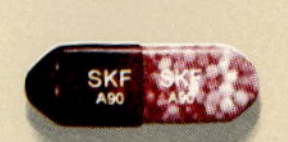 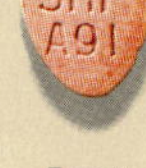 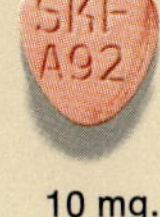

15 mg.   5 mg.   10 mg.

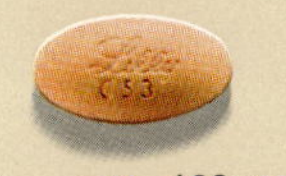

Darvon-N   100 mg.

Combined Identification Section

Demerol

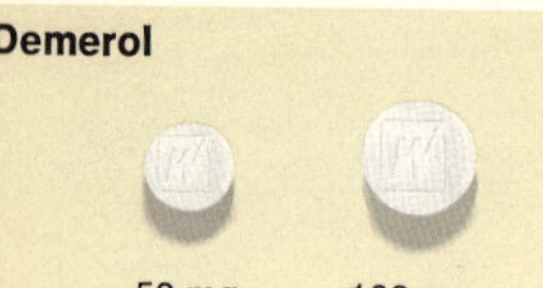

50 mg.　　100 mg.

Doriden

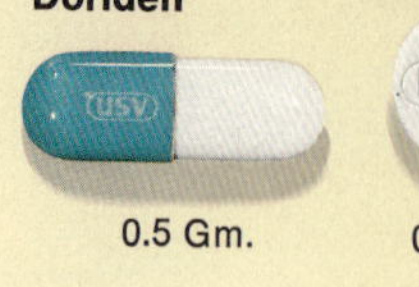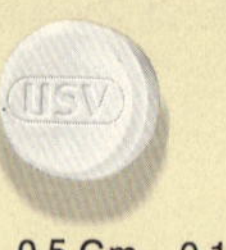

0.5 Gm.　　0.5 Gm.　0.125 Gm
　　　　　　　　　　0.25 Gm.

Desbutal

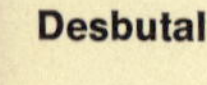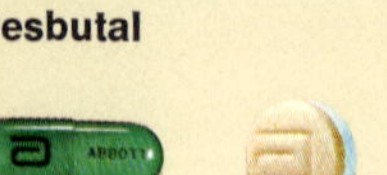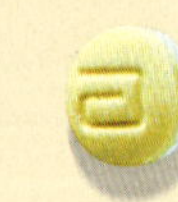

10　　15

Elavil

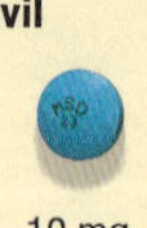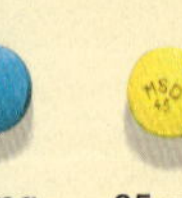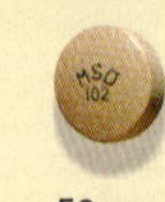

10 mg.　25 mg.　50 mg.

Desoxyn

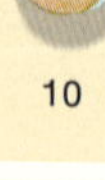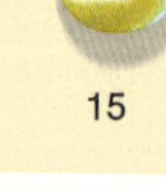

5 mg.　　10 mg.　　15 mg.

Equanil

200 mg.　　　400 mg.

Dexamyl

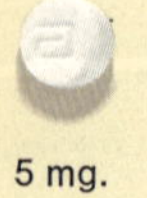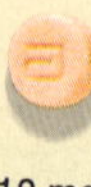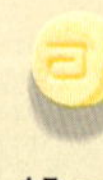

Also D91

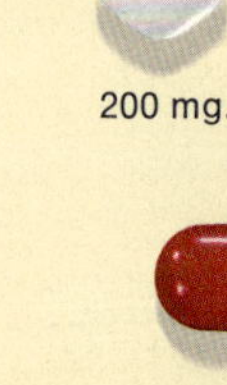

400 mg.

Dexedrine

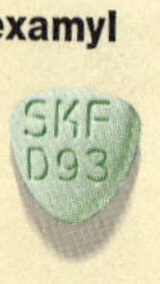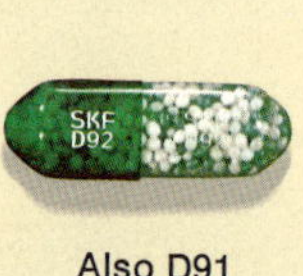

15 mg. (E14)

5 mg. (E12)
10 mg. (E13)

5 mg. (E19)

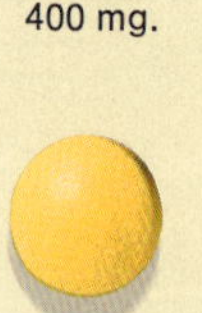

400 mg.
Wyseals

Dilaudid

Eskabarb

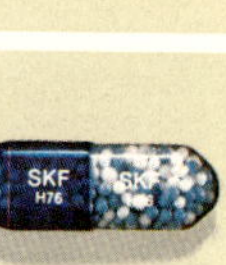

1½ gr. (H76)

Also: 1 gr. (H74)

Disipal

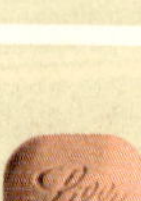

50 mg.

Eskalith

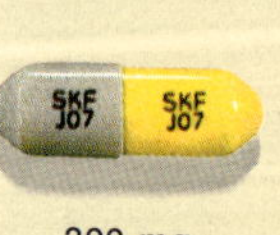

300 mg.

Diskets

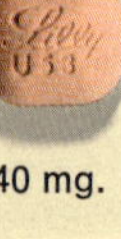

40 mg.

Eskaphen B

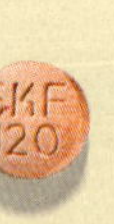

Dolophine HCl

10 mg.　　5 mg.

Etrafon

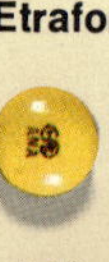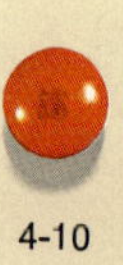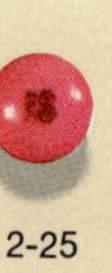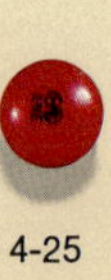

2-10　　4-10　　2-25　　4-25

Felsules

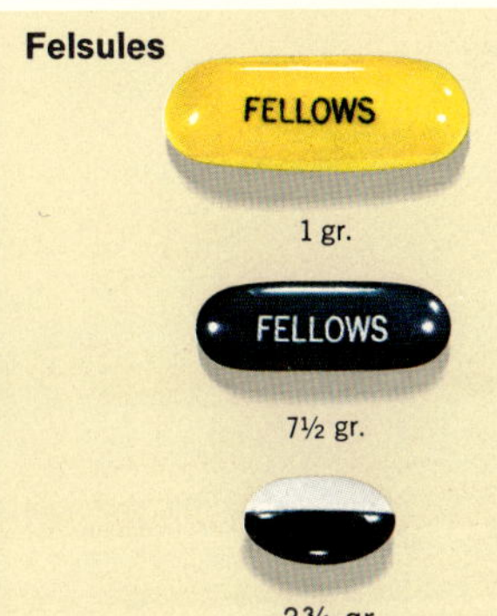

1 gr.

7½ gr.

3¾ gr.

Halabar

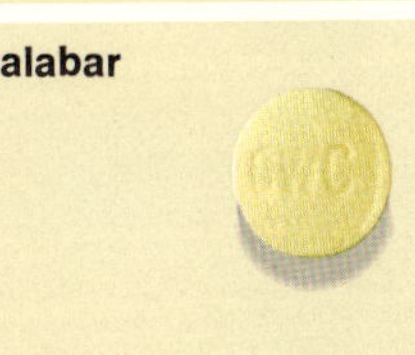

Haldol

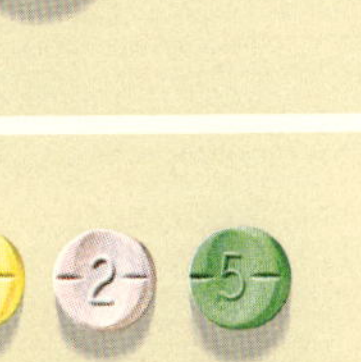

½ mg.   1 mg.   2 mg.   5 mg.

Kemadrin

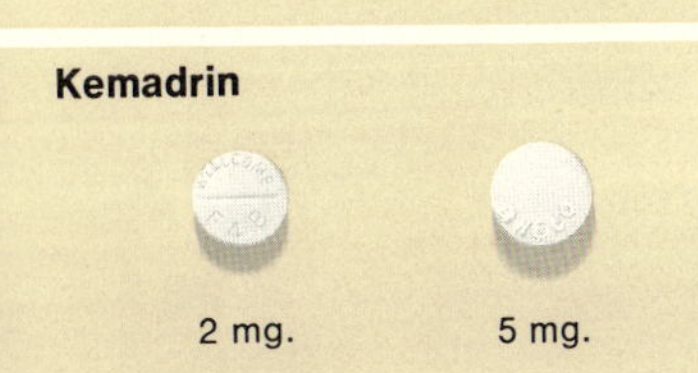

2 mg.   5 mg.

Kesso-Bamate

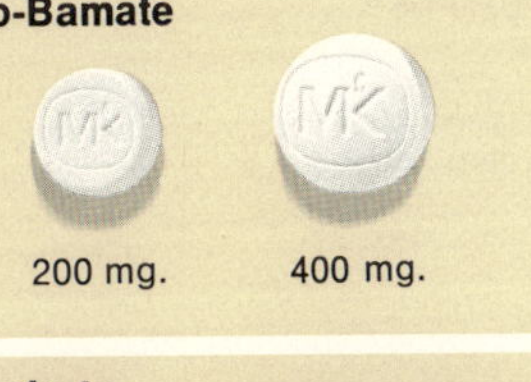

200 mg.   400 mg.

Kessodrate

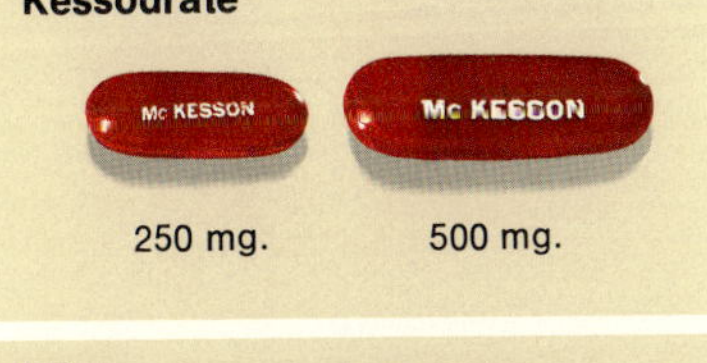

250 mg.   500 mg.

Librax

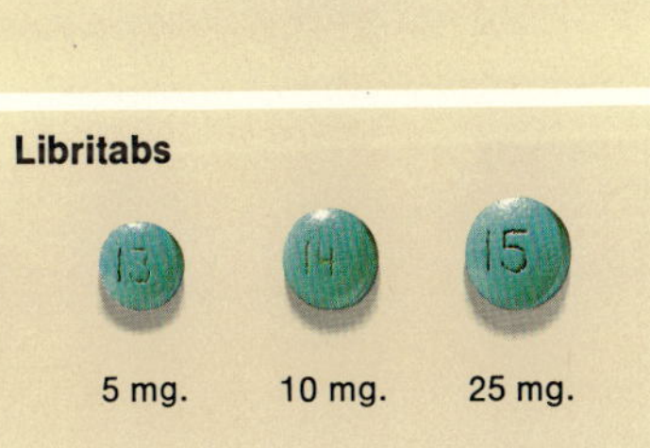

Libritabs

5 mg.   10 mg.   25 mg.

Librium

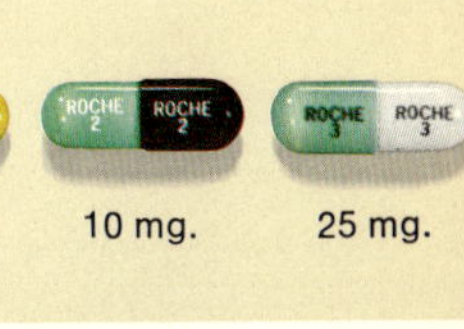

5 mg.   10 mg.   25 mg.

Lithane

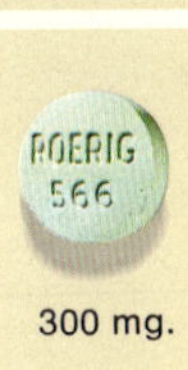

300 mg.

Lithonate

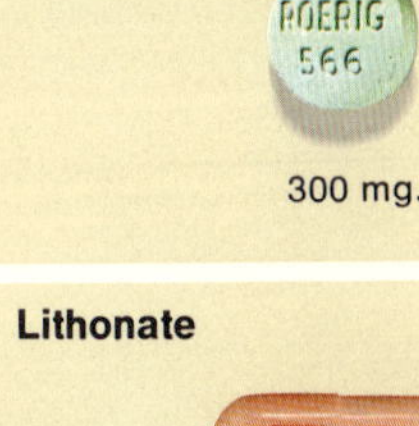

300 mg.

Luminal

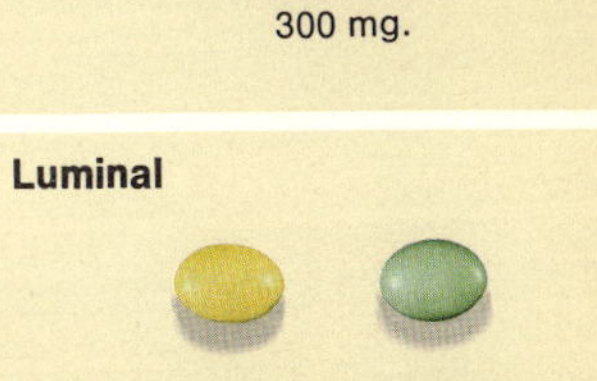

16 mg.   32 mg.

Marplan

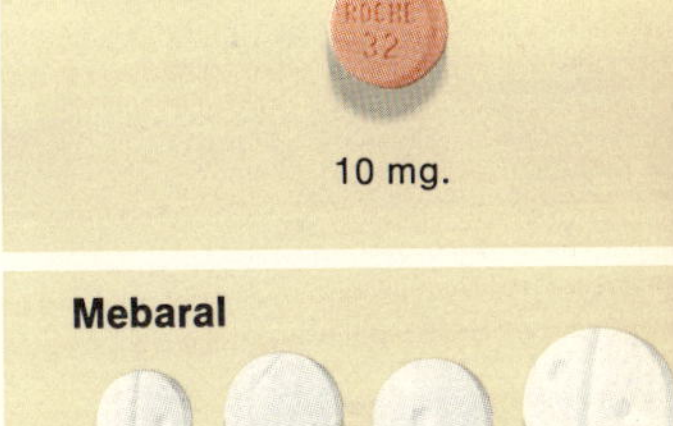

10 mg.

Mebaral

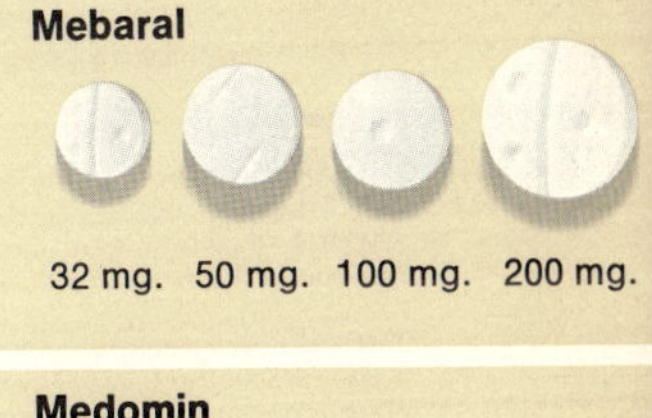

32 mg. 50 mg. 100 mg. 200 mg.

Medomin

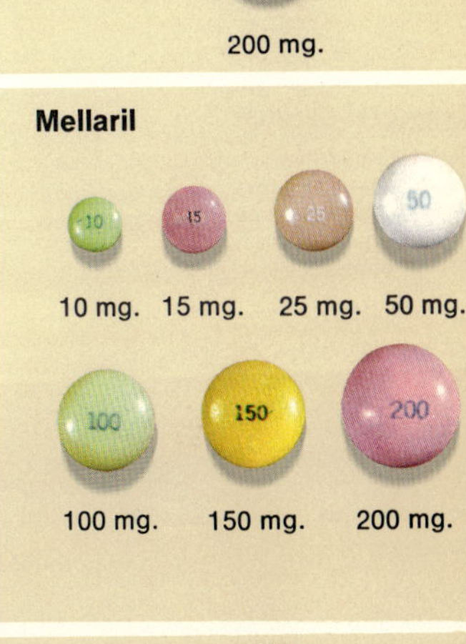

200 mg.

Mellaril

10 mg. 15 mg. 25 mg. 50 mg.

100 mg.   150 mg.   200 mg.

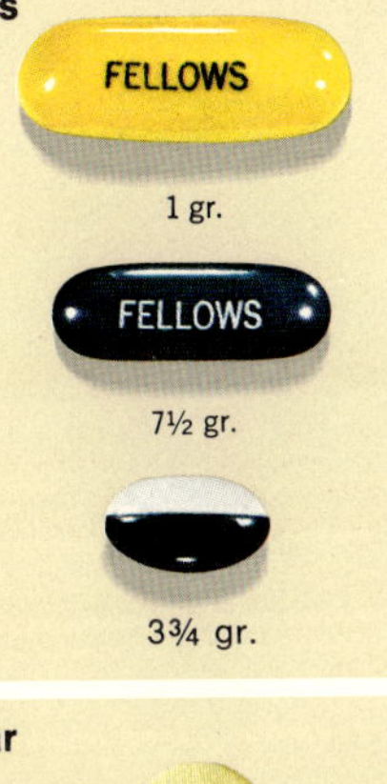
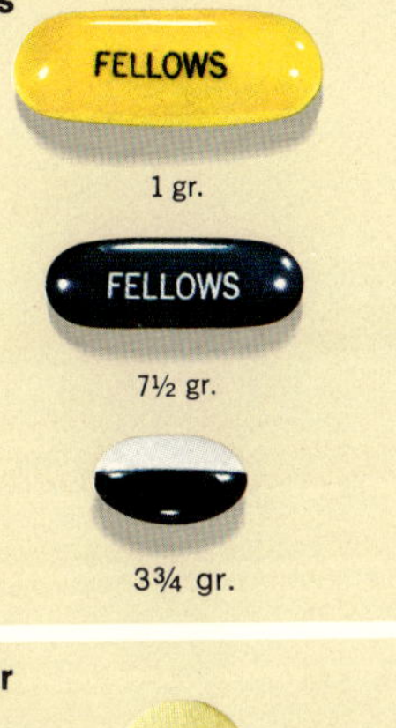
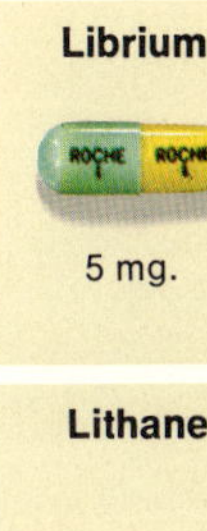

Combined Identification Section

Meprospan

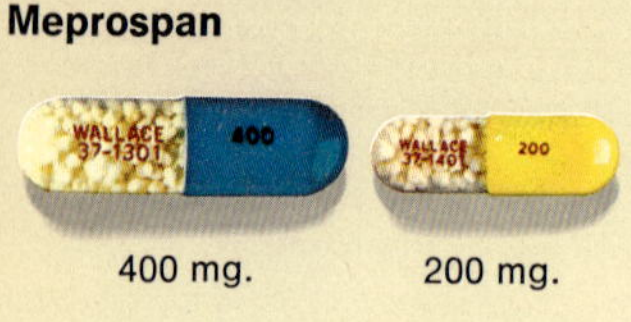

400 mg. 200 mg.

Meprotabs

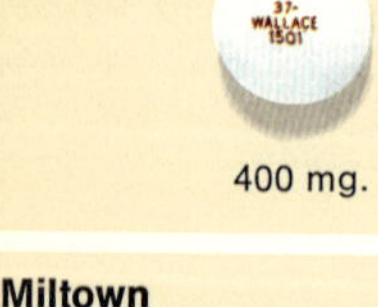

400 mg.

Miltown

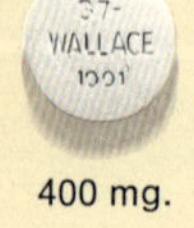 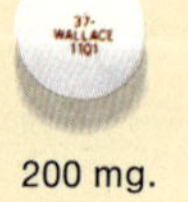

400 mg. 200 mg.

Nardil

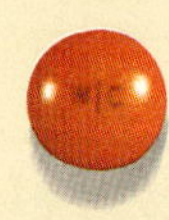

Navane

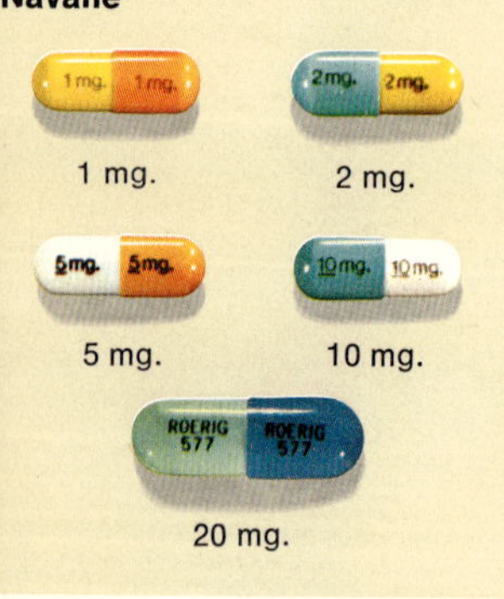

1 mg. 2 mg.

5 mg. 10 mg.

20 mg.

Nebralin

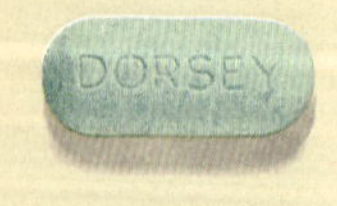

Nembutal Sodium

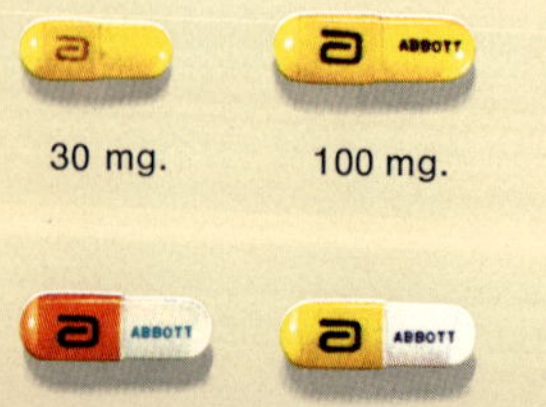

30 mg. 100 mg.

50 mg. 50 mg.

Niamid

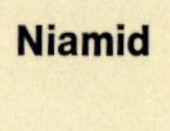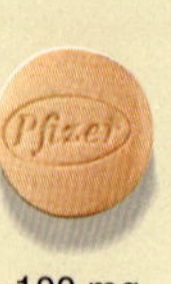

100 mg.

Noctec

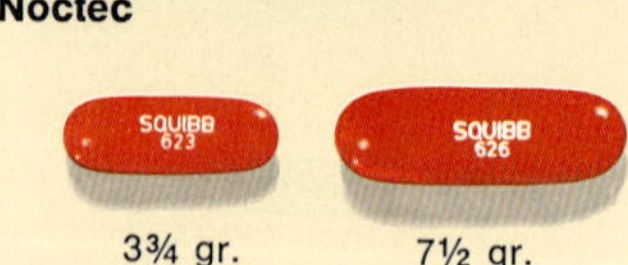

3¾ gr. 7½ gr.

Noludar

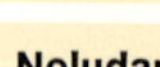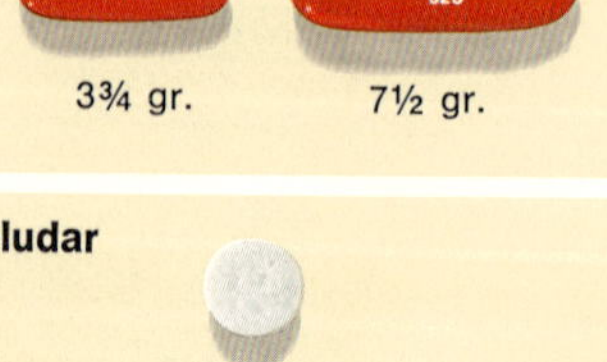

50 mg.

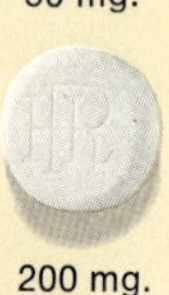

200 mg.

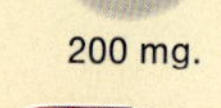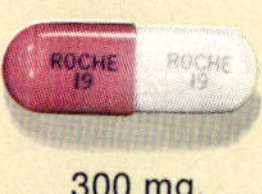

300 mg.

Norpramin

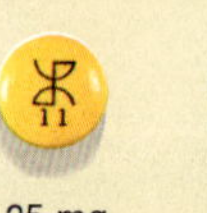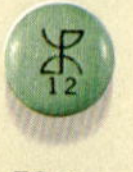

25 mg. 50 mg.

Optimil

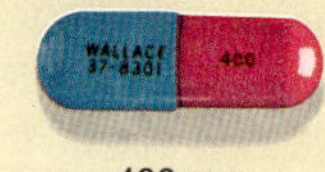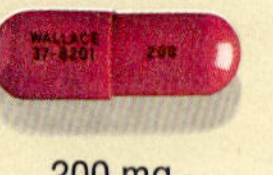

400 mg. 200 mg.

Pagitane HCl

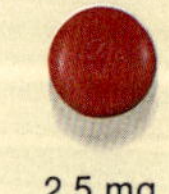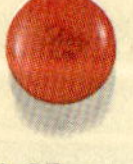

2.5 mg. 1.25 mg.

Parest

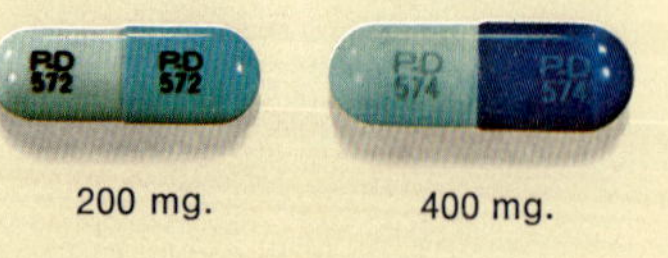

200 mg. 400 mg.

Parnate

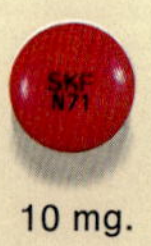

10 mg.

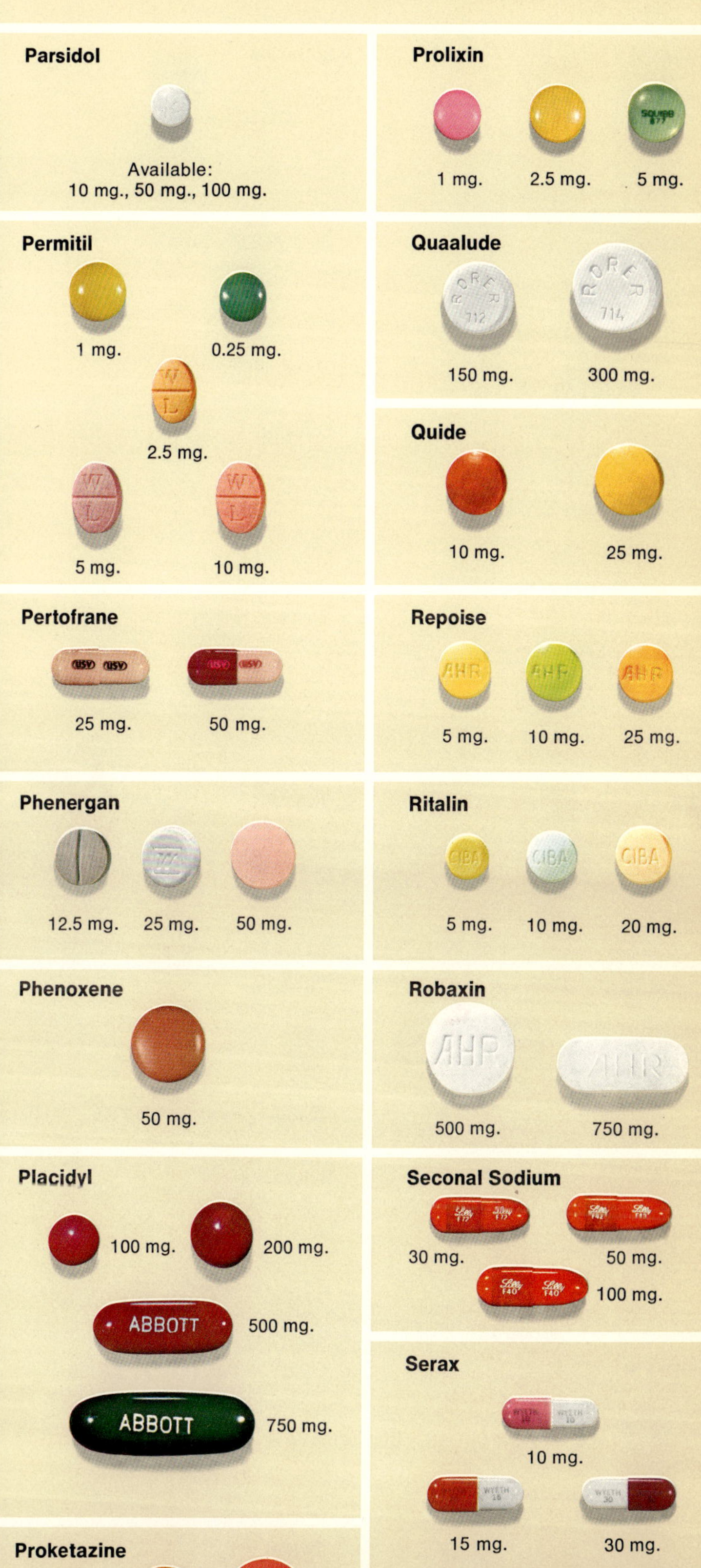

Parsidol
Available:
10 mg., 50 mg., 100 mg.

Permitil
1 mg.
0.25 mg.
2.5 mg.
5 mg.
10 mg.

Pertofrane
25 mg.
50 mg.

Phenergan
12.5 mg.
25 mg.
50 mg.

Phenoxene
50 mg.

Placidyl
100 mg.
200 mg.
ABBOTT
500 mg.
ABBOTT
750 mg.

Proketazine
12.5 mg.
25 mg.
50 mg.

Prolixin
1 mg.
2.5 mg.
5 mg.

Quaalude
150 mg.
300 mg.

Quide
10 mg.
25 mg.

Repoise
5 mg.
10 mg.
25 mg.

Ritalin
5 mg.
10 mg.
20 mg.

Robaxin
500 mg.
750 mg.

Seconal Sodium
30 mg.
50 mg.
100 mg.

Serax
10 mg.
15 mg.
30 mg.
15 mg.

Combined Identification Section

Serentil

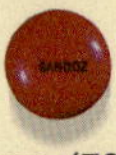

10 mg. (78-11)
25 mg. (78-12)
50 mg. (78-13)
100 mg. (78-14)

Stelazine

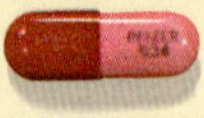

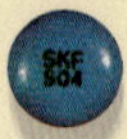

2 mg. (S04)
1 mg. (S03)
5 mg. (S06)
10 mg. (S07)

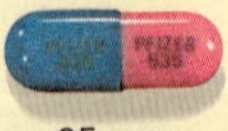

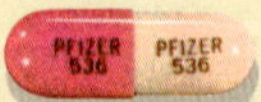

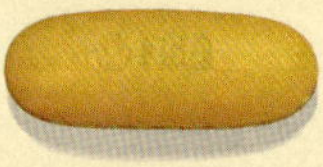

Sinequan

10 mg.

25 mg.

50 mg.

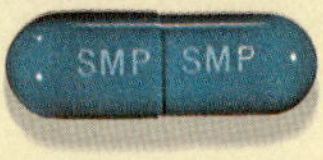

Stental Extentabs

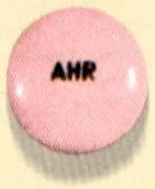

Suavitil

1 mg.

Solacen

350 mg.

Suvren

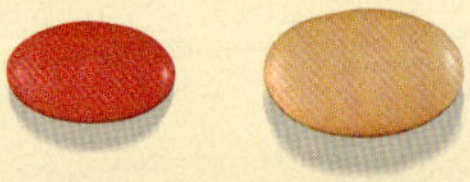

50 mg.   100 mg.

Solvets

Talwin

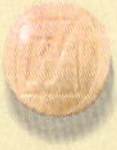

50 mg.

Somnafac

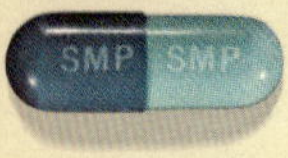

200 mg.   400 mg.
Somnafac Fourte

Taractan

10 mg.   25 mg.   50 mg.   100 mg.

Sopor

75 mg.   150 mg.   300 mg.

Thorazine

75 mg. (T64)   25 mg. (T74)

30 mg. (T63)   10 mg. (T73)
150 mg. (T66)   50 mg. (T76)
200 mg. (T67)   100 mg. (T77)
300 mg. (T69)   200 mg. (T79)

Sparine

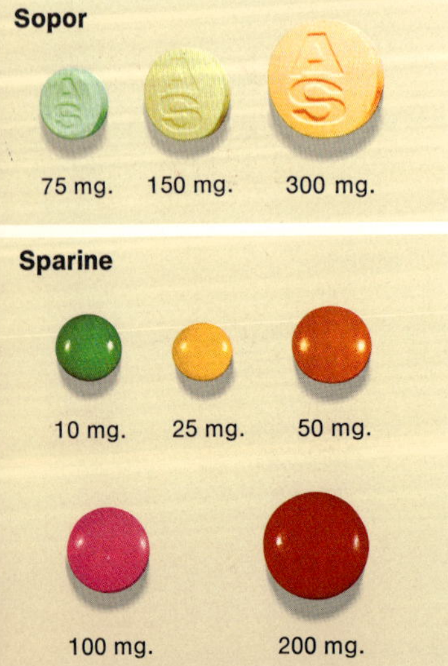

10 mg.   25 mg.   50 mg.

100 mg.   200 mg.

Tindal

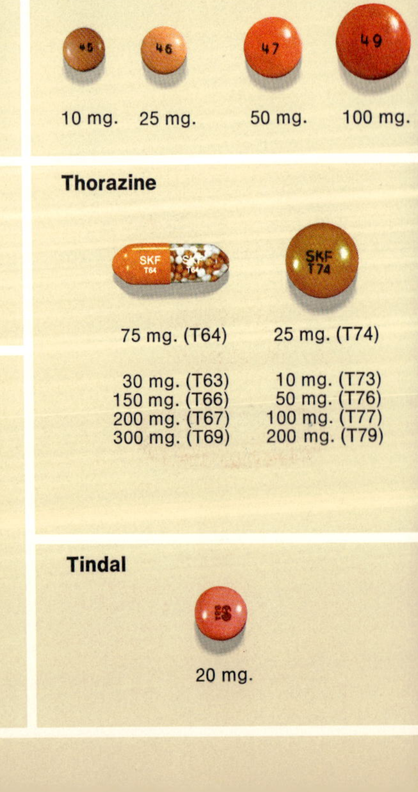

20 mg.

Tofranil

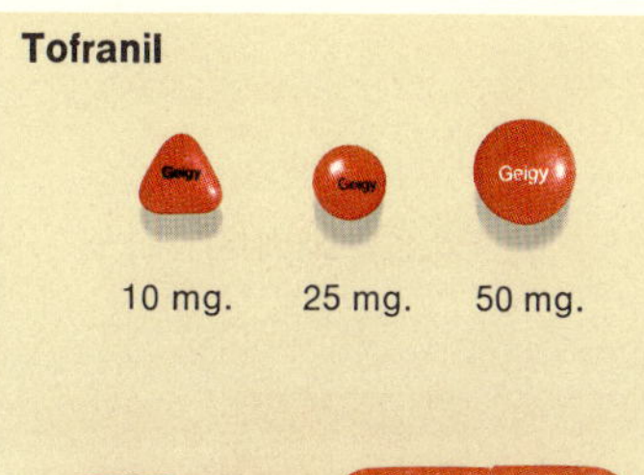

10 mg. 25 mg. 50 mg.

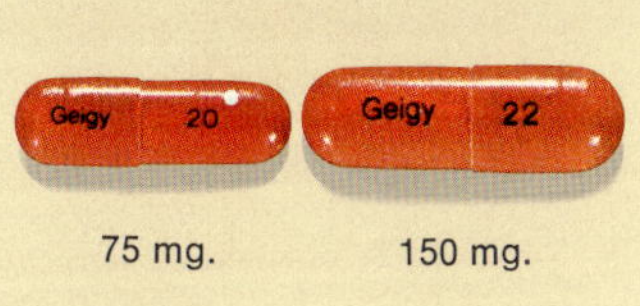

75 mg. 150 mg.

Trancopal

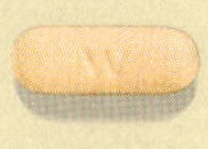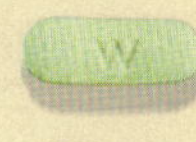

100 mg. 200 mg.

Triavil

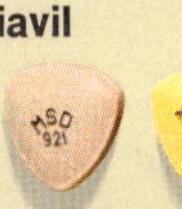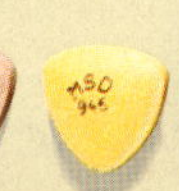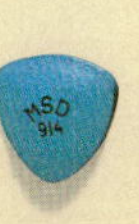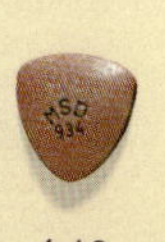

2-25 4-25 2-10 4-10

Trilafon

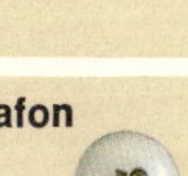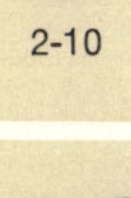

2 mg. 4 mg.

8 mg. 16 mg.

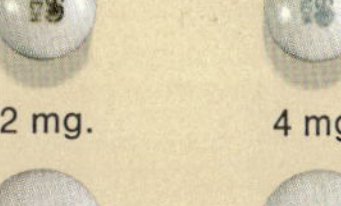

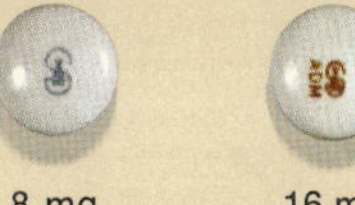

Trilafon Repetabs 8 mg.

Tuinal

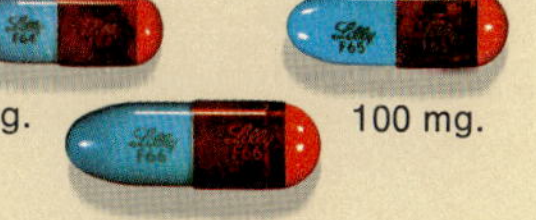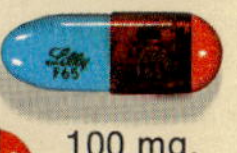

50 mg. 100 mg.

200 mg.

Tybatran

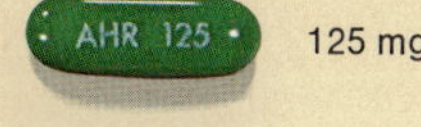 125 mg.

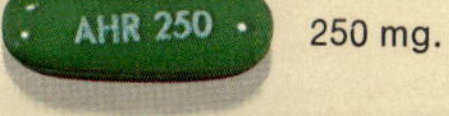 250 mg.

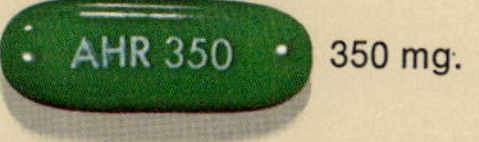 350 mg.

Ultran

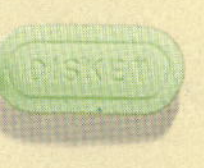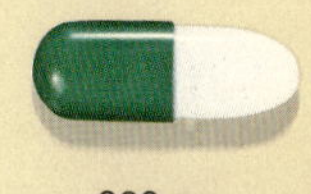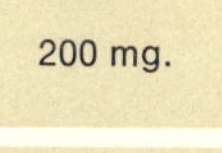

200 mg. 300 mg.

Valium

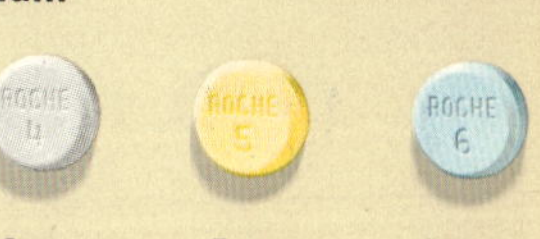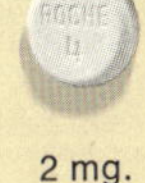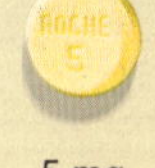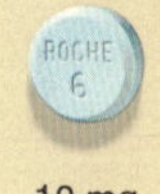

2 mg. 5 mg. 10 mg.

Valmid

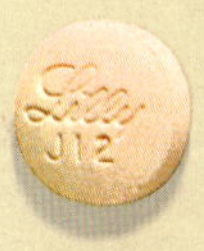

500 mg.

Vesprin

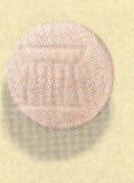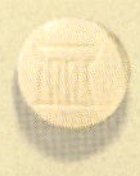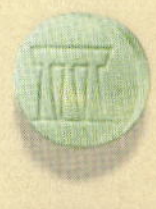

10 mg. 25 mg. 50 mg.

Vistaril

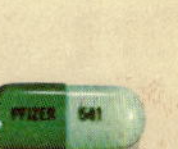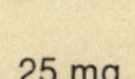

25 mg.

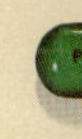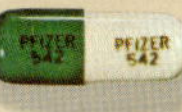

50 mg.

100 mg.

Vivactil

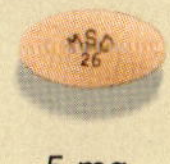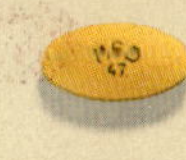

5 mg. 10 mg.

Every effort has been made to
reproduce these pharmaceutical
products faithfully; however,
these photographs should be
used only as a quick reference in
attempts to identify a particular
product. A chemical analysis
of any substance involved in a
case of drug overdosage should
always be obtained.

Capsules

Amytal Sodium

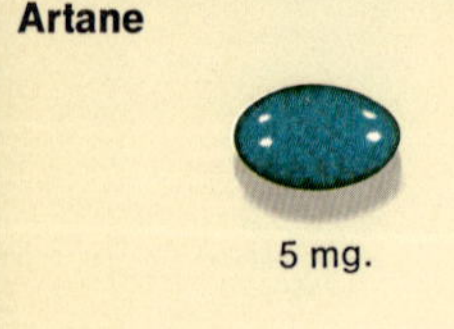

65 mg.   200 mg.

Artane

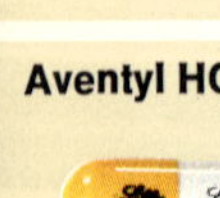

5 mg.

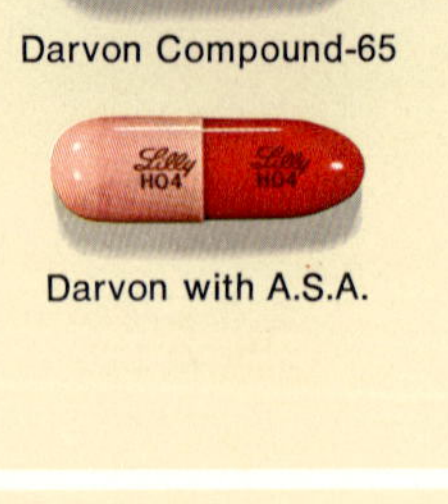

Darvon Compound-65

Darvon with A.S.A.

Aventyl HCl

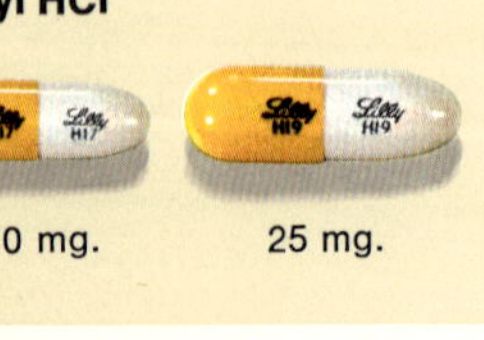

10 mg.   25 mg.

Desbutal

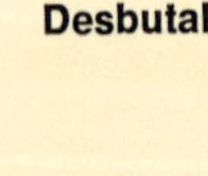

Benadryl

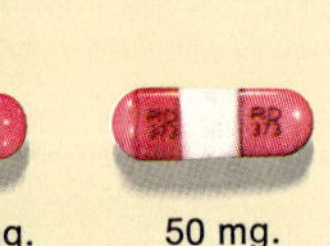

25 mg.   50 mg.

Dexamyl

Also D91

Benzedrine

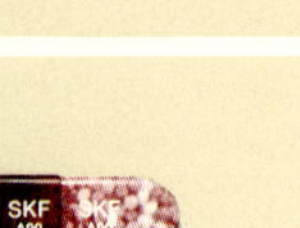

15 mg.

Dexedrine

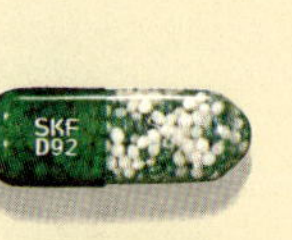

15 mg. (E14)

5 mg. (E12)
10 mg. (E13)

Buticaps

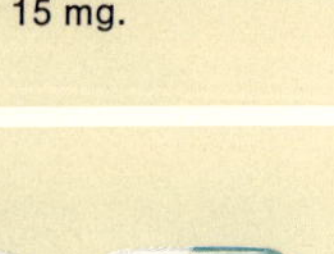

¼ gr.   ½ gr.

Doriden

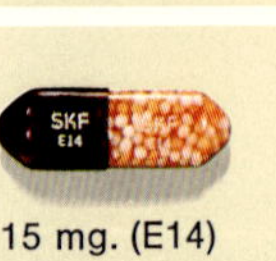

0.5 Gm.

Compazine

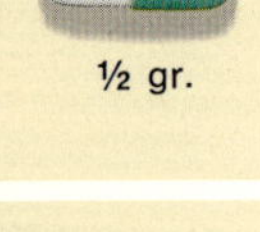

15 mg. (C46)   10 mg. (C44)
               30 mg. (C47)
               75 mg. (C49)

Equanil

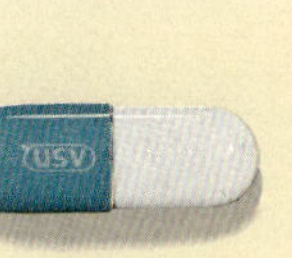

400 mg.

Darvon

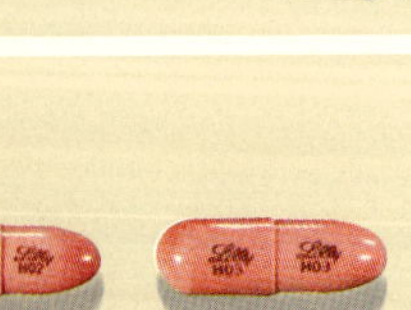

32 mg.   65 mg.

Eskabarb

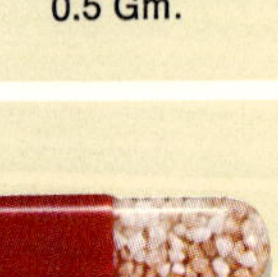

1½ gr. (H·76)
Also: 1 gr. (H74)

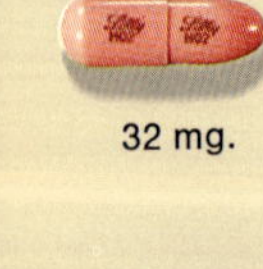
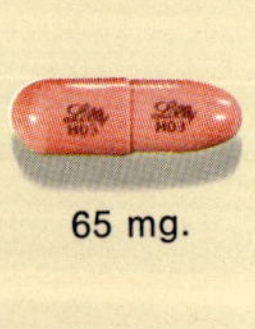

Darvon Compound

Eskalith

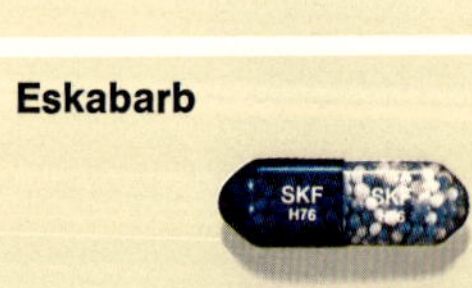

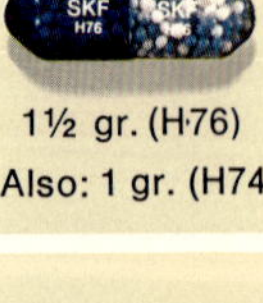
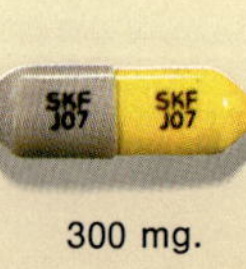

300 mg.

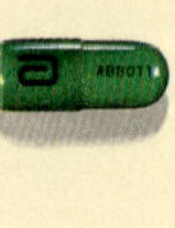
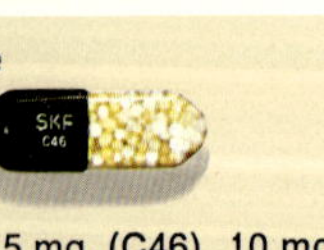

Felsules

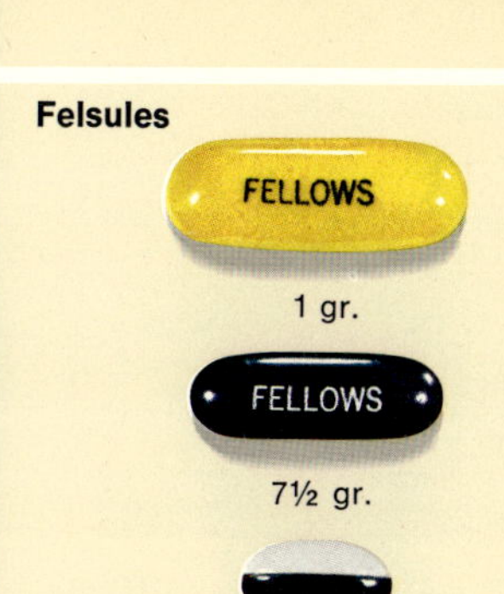

1 gr.

7½ gr.

3¾ gr.

Nembutal Sodium

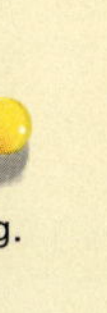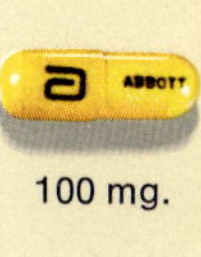

30 mg.

100 mg.

50 mg.

50 mg.

Kessodrate

250 mg.

500 mg.

Noctec

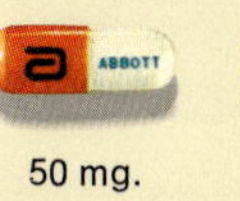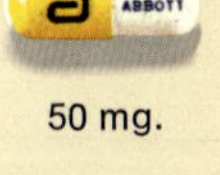

3¾ gr.

7½ gr.

Librax

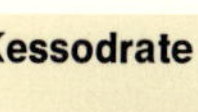

Noludar

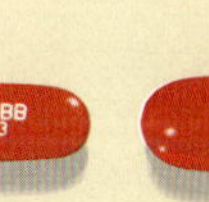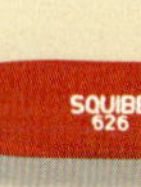

300 mg.

Librium

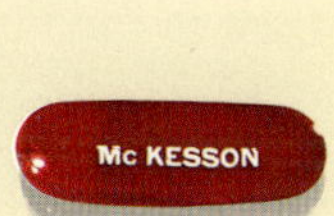

5 mg.

10 mg.

25 mg.

Optimil

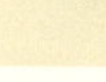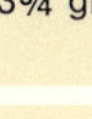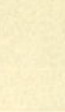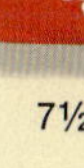

400 mg.

200 mg.

Lithonate

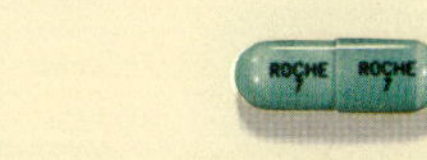

300 mg.

Parest

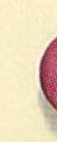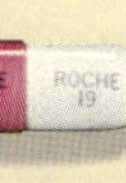

200 mg.

400 mg.

Meprospan

400 mg.

200 mg.

Pertofrane

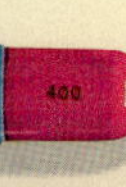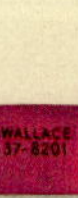

25 mg.

50 mg.

Navane

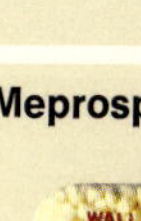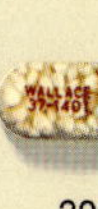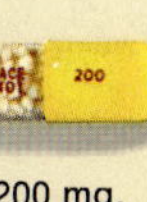

1 mg.

2 mg.

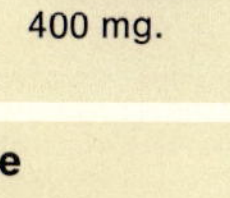

5 mg.

10 mg.

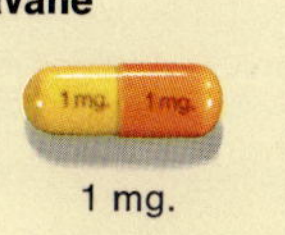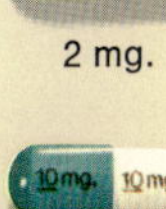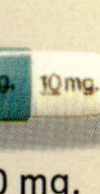

20 mg.

Placidyl

 500 mg.

 750 mg.

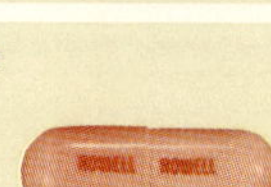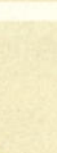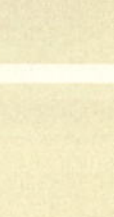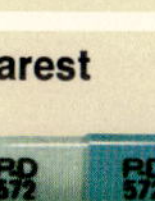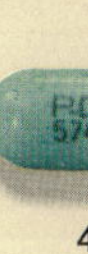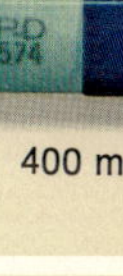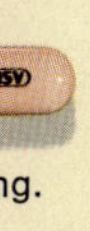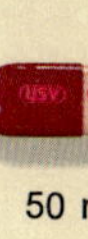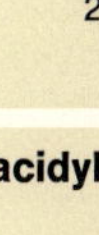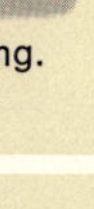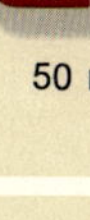

Capsules

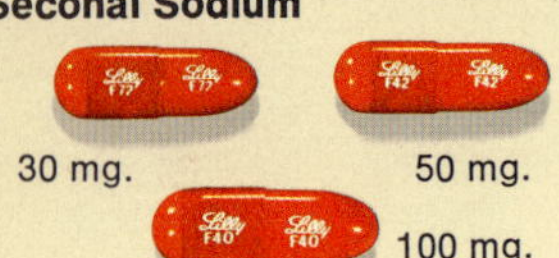

Seconal Sodium

30 mg.

50 mg.

100 mg.

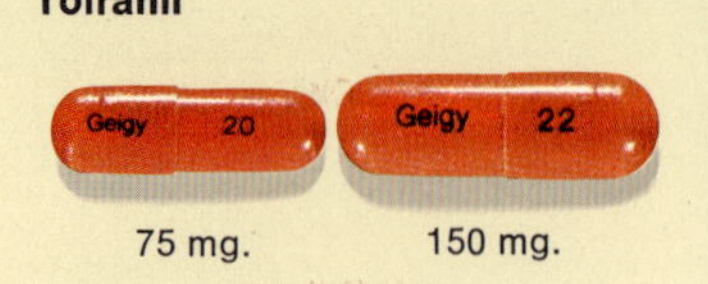

Tofranil

75 mg.

150 mg.

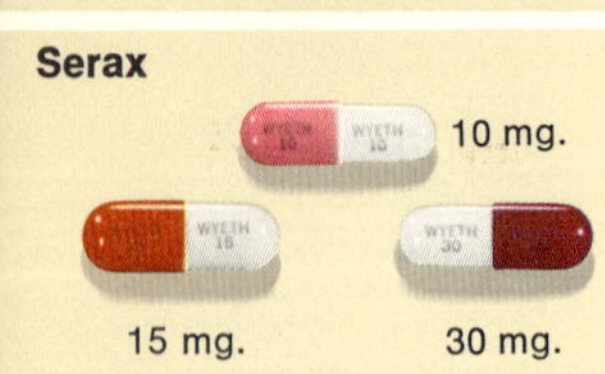

Serax

10 mg.

15 mg.

30 mg.

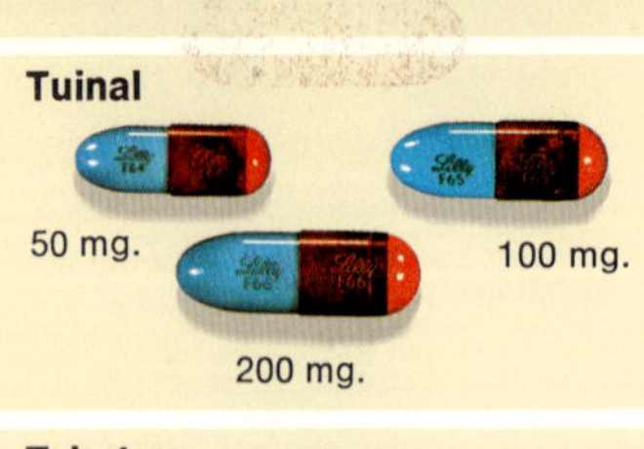

Tuinal

50 mg.

100 mg.

200 mg.

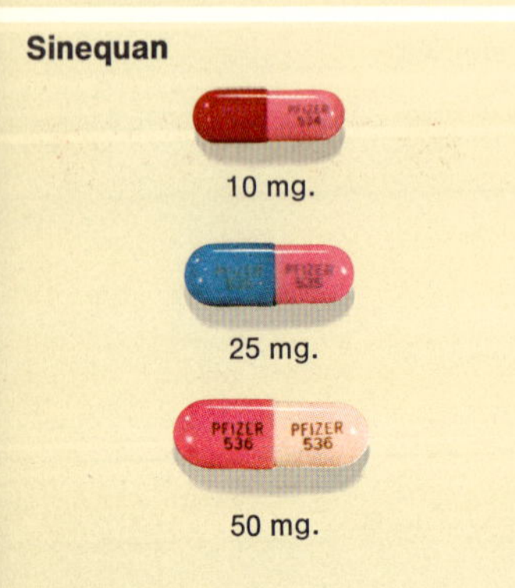

Sinequan

10 mg.

25 mg.

50 mg.

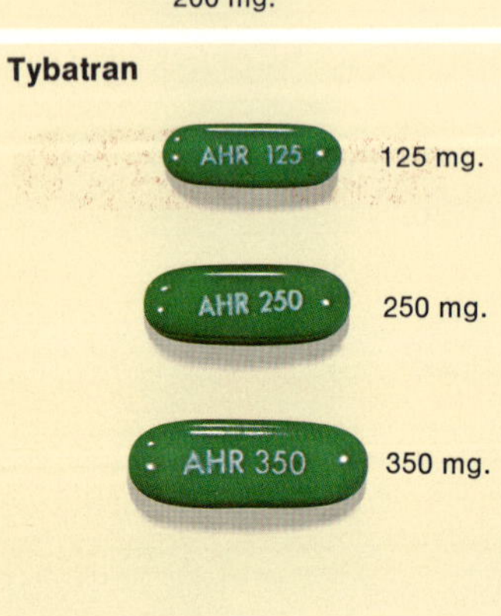

Tybatran

125 mg.

250 mg.

350 mg.

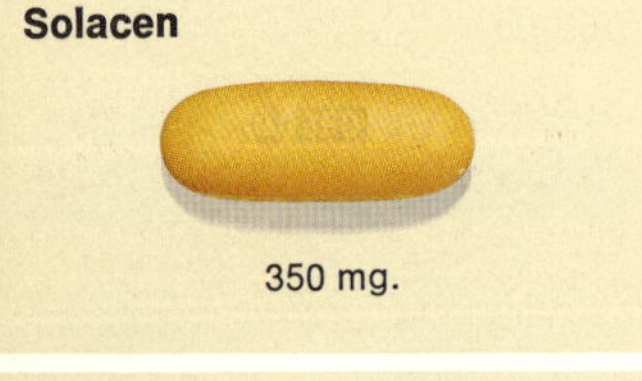

Solacen

350 mg.

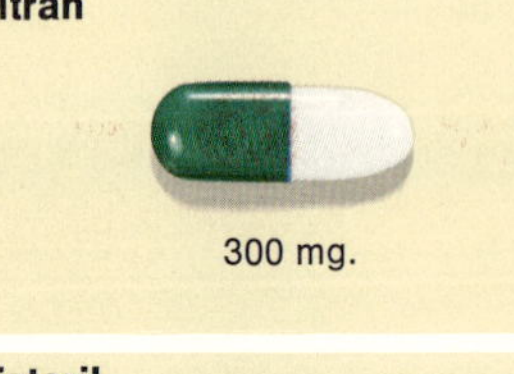

Ultran

300 mg.

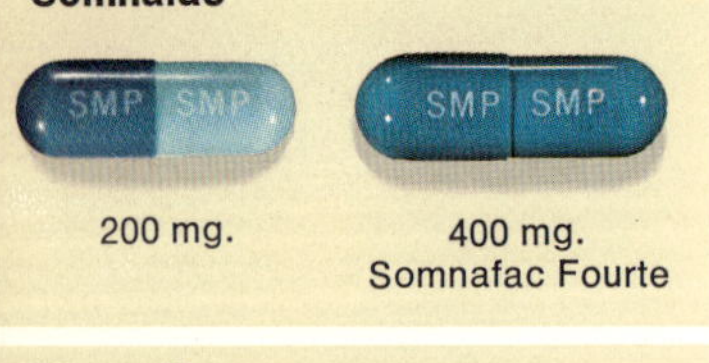

Somnafac

200 mg.

400 mg.
Somnafac Fourte

Thorazine

75 mg. (T64)

30 mg. (T63)   200 mg. (T67)
150 mg. (T66)   300 mg. (T69)

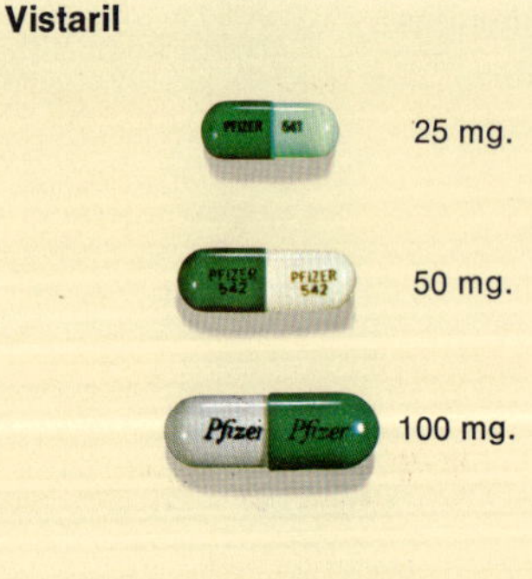

Vistaril

25 mg.

50 mg.

100 mg.

Tablets (white)

Akineton 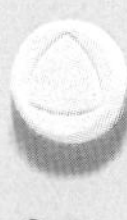 2 mg.	**Equanil** 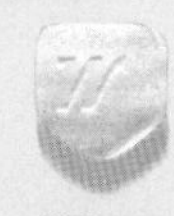 200 mg. 400 mg.
Artane 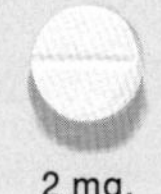 2 mg. 5 mg.	**Haldol** 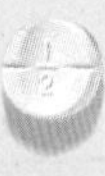 ½ mg.
Cogentin 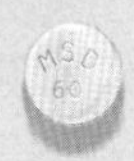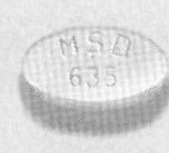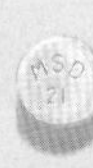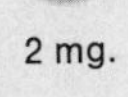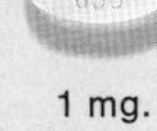 2 mg. 1 mg. 0.5 mg.	**Kemadrin**  2 mg. 5 mg.
Dartal 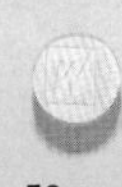 5 mg.	**Kesso-Bamate** 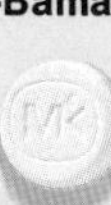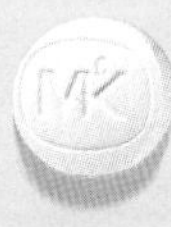 200 mg. 400 mg.
Demerol 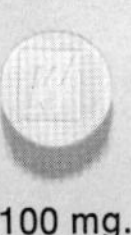 50 mg. 100 mg.	**Mebaral**  32 mg. 50 mg. 100 mg. 200 mg.
Desoxyn  5 mg.	**Medomin** 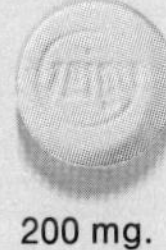 200 mg.
Dilaudid 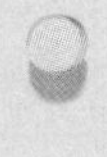	**Mellaril** 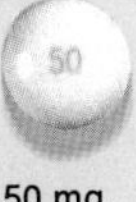 50 mg.
Dolophine HCl 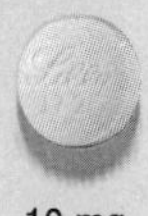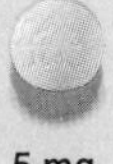 10 mg. 5 mg.	**Meprotabs** 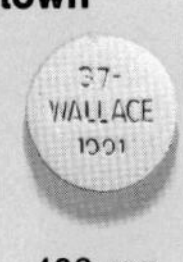 400 mg.
Doriden 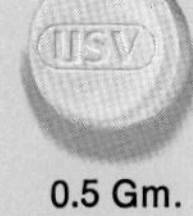 0.5 Gm. 0.125 Gm. 0.25 Gm.	**Miltown** 400 mg. 200 mg.

Tablets (white)

Noludar

 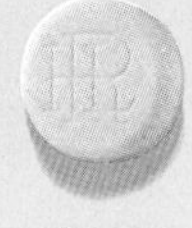

50 mg.   200 mg.

Solvets

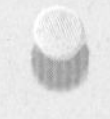

Parsidol

Available:
10 mg., 50 mg., 100 mg.

Suavitil

1 mg.

Phenergan

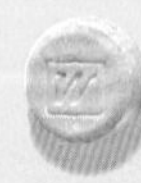

25 mg.

Trilafon

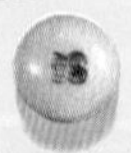 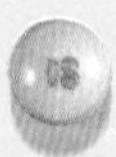

2 mg.   4 mg.

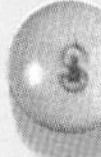 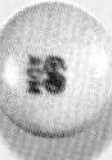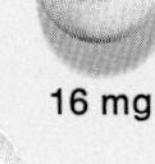

8 mg.   16 mg.

Trilafon Repetabs 8 mg.

Quaalude

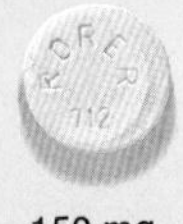

150 mg.   300 mg.

Robaxin

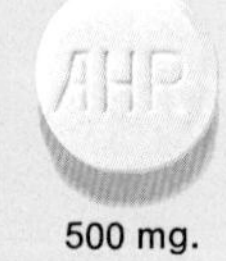  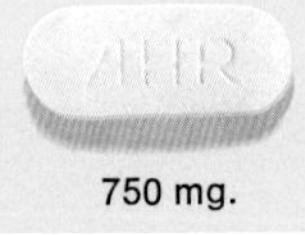

500 mg.   750 mg.

Valium

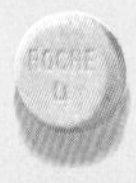

2 mg.

Tablets (colored)

Adipex Ty-Med

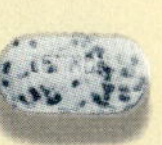

Desbutal

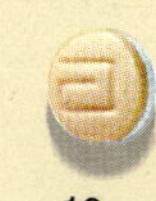
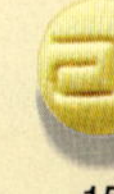

10   15

Amytal

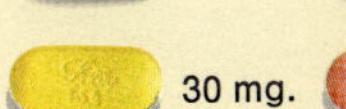

15 mg.   50 mg.

30 mg.   100 mg.

Desoxyn

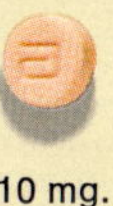
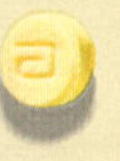

10 mg.   15 mg.

Atarax

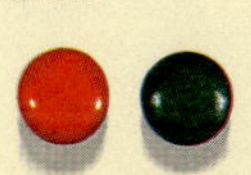
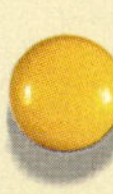
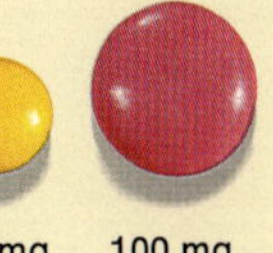

10 mg.   25 mg.   50 mg.   100 mg.

Dexamyl

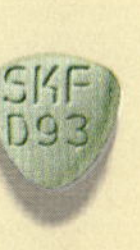

Benzedrine

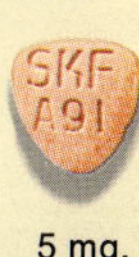

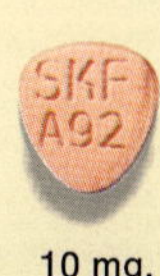

5 mg.   10 mg.

Dexedrine

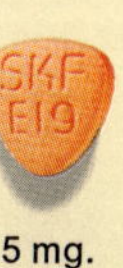

5 mg.

Butisol Sodium

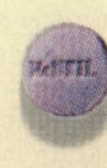
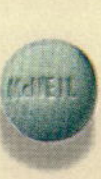
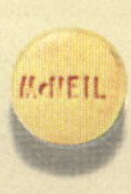
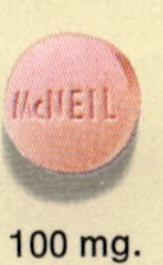

15 mg.   30 mg.   50 mg.   100 mg.

Disipal

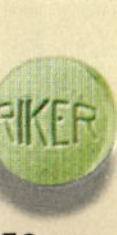

50 mg.

Compazine

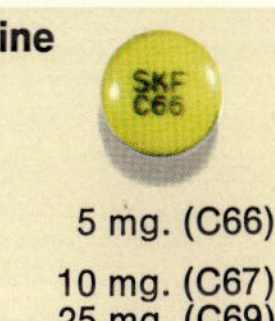

5 mg. (C66)
10 mg. (C67)
25 mg. (C69)

Diskets

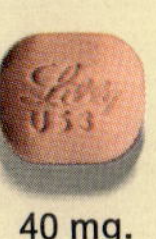

40 mg.

Dartal

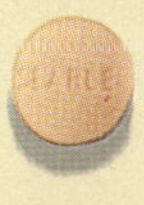

10 mg.

Elavil

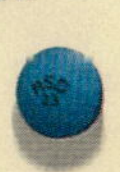
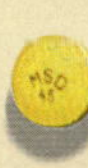
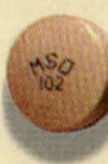

10 mg.   25 mg.   50 mg.

Darvon

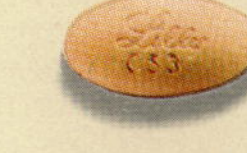

Darvon-N with A.S.A.

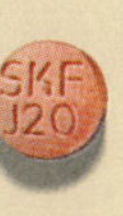

Darvon-N   100 mg.

Equanil

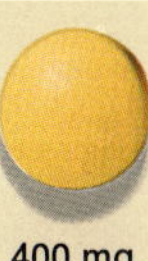

400 mg.
Wyseals

Eskaphen B

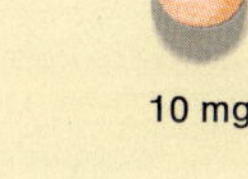

Tablets (colored)

Etrafon

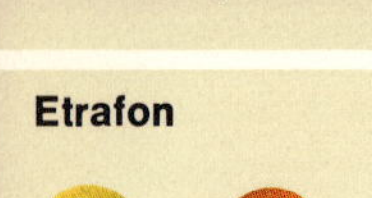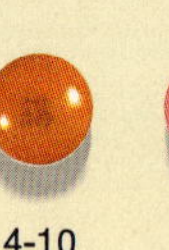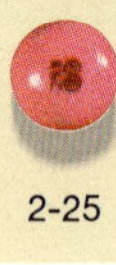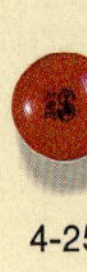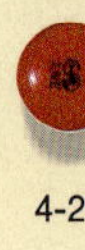

2-10   4-10   2-25   4-25

Nardil

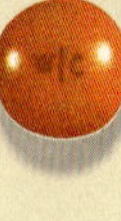

Halabar

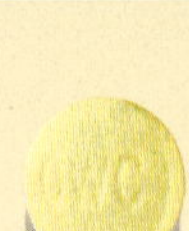

Nebralin

Haldol

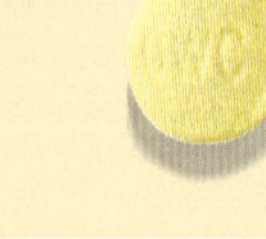

1 mg.   2 mg.   5 mg.

Niamid

100 mg.

Libritabs

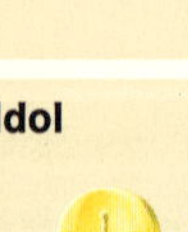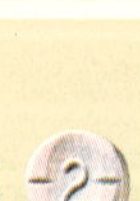

5 mg.   10 mg.   25 mg.

Norpramin

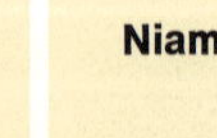

25 mg.   50 mg.

Lithane

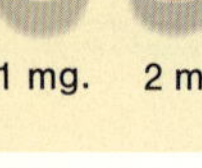

300 mg.

Pagitane HCl

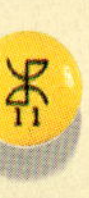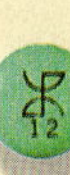

2.5 mg.   1.25 mg.

Luminal

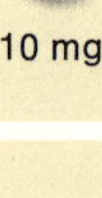

16 mg.   32 mg.

Parnate

10 mg.

Marplan

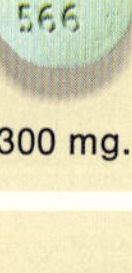

10 mg.

Permitil

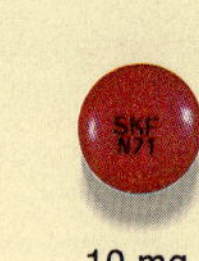

1 mg.   0.25 mg.

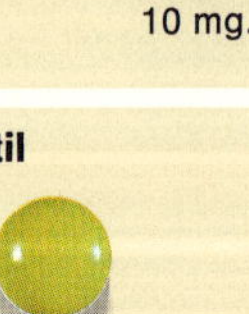

2.5 mg.

Mellaril

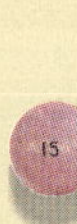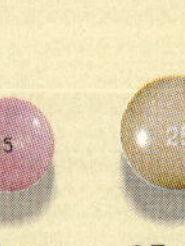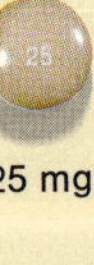

10 mg. 15 mg. 25 mg.

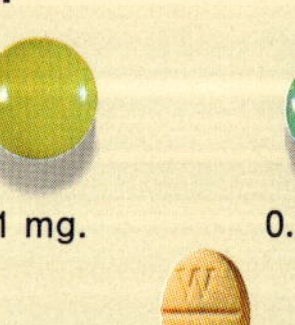

5 mg.   10 mg.

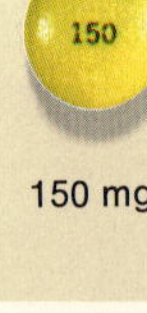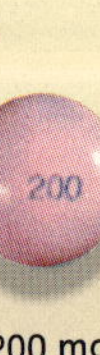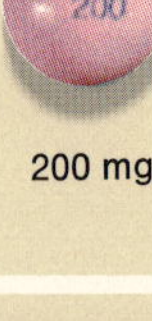

100 mg. 150 mg. 200 mg.

Phenergan

12.5 mg.   50 mg.

Phenoxene

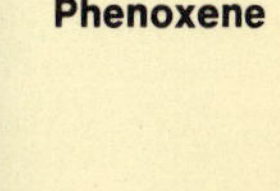

50 mg.

Sopor

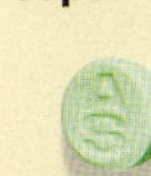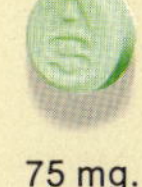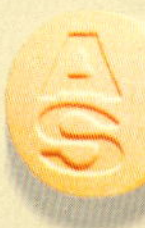

75 mg.   150 mg.   300 mg.

Placidyl

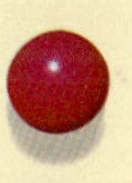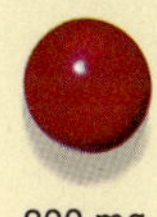

100 mg.   200 mg.

Sparine

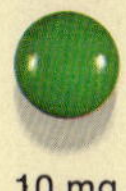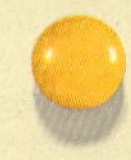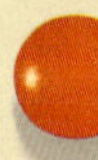

10 mg.   25 mg.   50 mg.

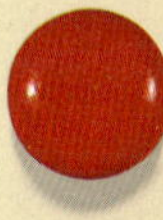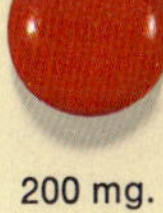

100 mg.   200 mg.

Proketazine

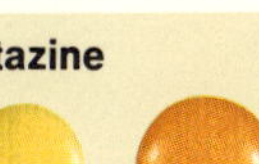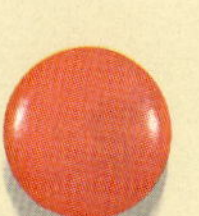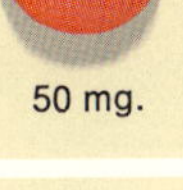

12.5 mg.   25 mg.   50 mg.

Prolixin

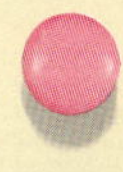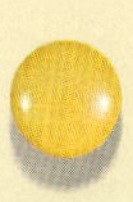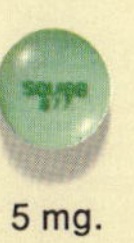

1 mg.   2.5 mg.   5 mg.

Stelazine

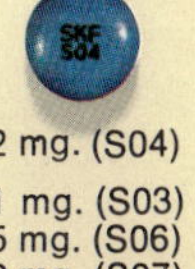

2 mg. (S04)

1 mg. (S03)
5 mg. (S06)
10 mg. (S07)

Quide

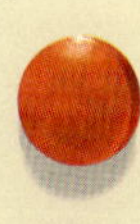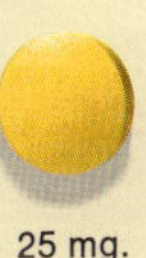

10 mg.   25 mg.

Stental Extentabs

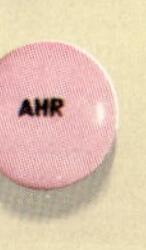

Repoise

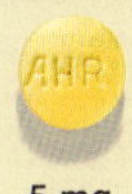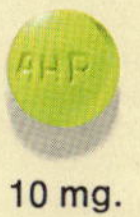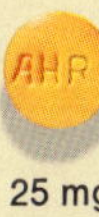

5 mg.   10 mg.   25 mg.

Suvren

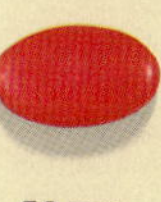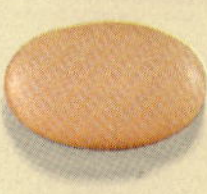

50 mg.   100 mg.

Ritalin

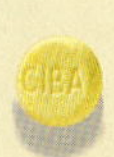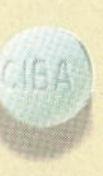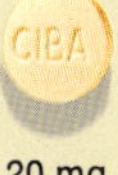
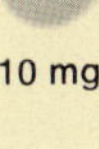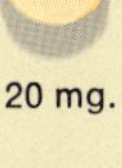

5 mg.   10 mg.   20 mg.

Talwin

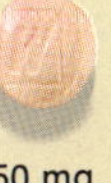

50 mg.

Serax

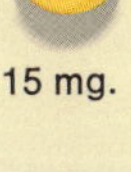

15 mg.

Taractan

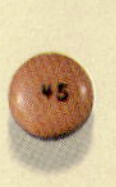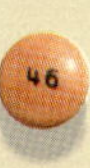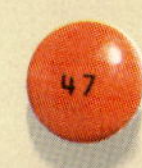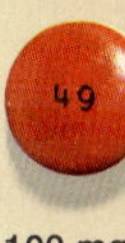

10 mg.   25 mg.   50 mg.   100 mg.

Serentil

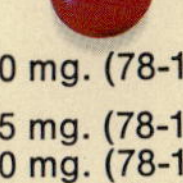

10 mg. (78-11)

25 mg. (78-12)
50 mg. (78-13)
100 mg. (78-14)

Thorazine

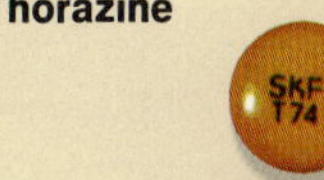

25 mg. (T74)

10 mg. (T73)   100 mg. (T77)
50 mg. (T76)   200 mg. (T79)

Tablets (colored)

Tindal

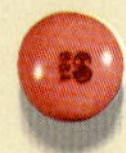

20 mg.

Tofranil

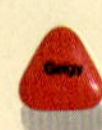 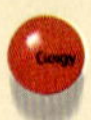 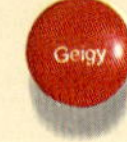

10 mg.   25 mg.   50 mg.

Trancopal

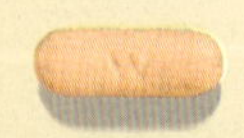 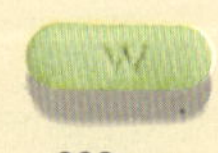

100 mg.   200 mg.

Triavil

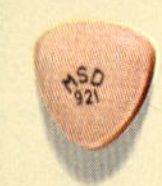 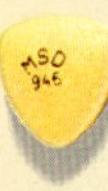 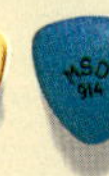 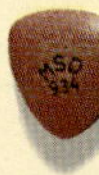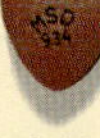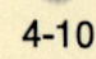

2-25   4-25   2-10   4-10

Ultran

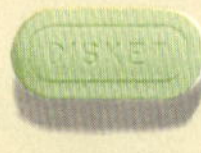

200 mg.

Valium

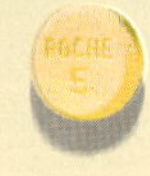 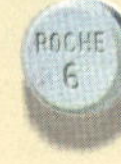

5 mg.   10 mg.

Valmid

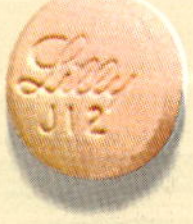

500 mg.

Vesprin

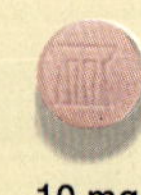 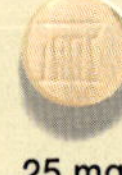 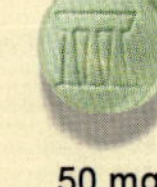

10 mg.   25 mg.   50 mg.

Vivactil

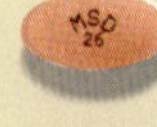 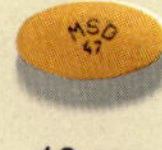

5 mg.   10 mg.

Poison Control Centers

This list of Poison Control Centers is based on information filed with the National Clearinghouse for Poison Control Centers. It includes those facilities which provide information to medical personnel on a continual basis about the treatment of patients who have ingested harmful amounts of potentially dangerous drugs or poisonous substances.

→

Alabama

State Coordinator
State Department of Public Health   265-2341
Montgomery 36104

Anniston   Poison Control Center, Anniston Memorial   237-5421
Hospital Pharmacy Department   Ext. 382
400 East 10th Street, P.O. Box 370 36201

Auburn   Poison Control Center, School of Pharmacy,   826-4740
Auburn University 36830

Birmingham   Poison Control Center, Children's Hospital   323-8901
1601 6th Avenue, South 35233

Dothan   Poison Control Center   794-3131
Southeast Alabama General Hospital 36301   Ext. 521

Florence   Poison Control Center   764-8321
Eliza Coffee Memorial Hospital   Ext. 206
600 West Alabama Street 35630

Gadsden   Poison Control Center   492-1240
Baptist Memorial Hospital   Ext. 206
1007 Goodyear Avenue 35903

Mobile   Poison Control Center   473-0341
Mobile General Hospital   Ext. 243
St. Anthony & Broad Streets 36603

Alaska

State Coordinator
State Department of Health and Welfare   586-6311
Juneau 99801

Anchorage   Poison Control Center   279-6661
Alaska Native Medical Center   Ext. 208
Public Health Service, Box 7-741 95501   209, 210, 211

Fairbanks   Poison Control Center   456-6655
Fairbanks Community Hospital   Ext. 35
119 North Cushman 99701

Juneau   Poison Control Center   586-2611
Greater Juneau Borough Hospital
419 6th Street 99801

Ketchikan   Poison Information Center   225-5171
Ketchikan General Hospital   Ext. 31
3100 Tongass Avenue 99901

Mt. Edgecumbe   Poison Control Center   966-8347
Alaska Native Hospital
Public Health Service 99835

Arizona

State Coordinator
University of Arizona, Tucson 85721   884-0111

Douglas   Poison Control Center, Douglas Hospital   364-2421
610 9th Street 85607

Flagstaff   Poison Control Center, Flagstaff Hospital   744-5233
1215 North Beaver Street 86001

Ganado   Poison Control Center, Project Hope   755-3411
Sage Memorial Hospital, Box 457 86505

Kingman   Poison Control Center   753-6132
Mohave General Hospital   Ext. 245
301 West Beale 86441   265

Nogales   Poison Control Center   287-2771
St. Joseph's Hospital   Ext. 94
Target Range Road
P.O. Box 1809 85621

Phoenix   Poison Control Center   252-6611
Good Samaritan Hospital   Ext. 221
1033 East McDowell Road 85006

Poison Control Center   272-6611
Maricopa County General Hospital   Ext. 317
3435 West Durango 85009

Poison Control Center, Memorial Hospital   252-5911
1200 South 5th Avenue 85003

Poison Control Center, St. Joseph's Hospital   277-6611
350 West Thomas Road 85013   Ext. 581

Poison Control Center   258-7373
St. Luke's Hospital Medical Center   Ext. 291
525 North 18th Street 85006

Stamford	Poison Control Center, Stamford Hospital Shelburne Road at West Broad Street 06902	327-1234 Ext. 333
Waterbury	Poison Control Center, St. Mary's Hospital 56 Franklin Street 06702	756-8351 Ext. 210

Delaware

Wilmington	Poison Information Service 501 West 14th Street 19899	655-3389

District of Columbia

Washington	Poison Control Center, Children's Hospital 13th & W Streets, North West 20009	835-4080 or 4081

Florida

	State Coordinator Dept. of Health and Rehabilitative Services Jacksonville 32201	354-3961
Apalachicola	Poison Control Center George E. Weems Memorial Hospital Franklin Square, Box 610 32320	653-3311
Bartow	Poison Control Center Polk General Hospital 2010 E. Georgia Street, P.O. Box 81 33830	533-1111 Ext. 237
Bradenton	Poison Control Center Manatee Memorial Hospital 206 2nd Street 33505	746-5111 Ext. 466
Daytona Beach	Poison Control Center Halifax District Hospital Clyde Morris Boulevard 32015	255-4411 Ext. 256
Fort Lauderdale	Poison Control Center Broward General Hospital 1600 South Andrews Avenue 33316	525-5411 Ext. 513
Fort Myers	Poison Control Center Lee Memorial Hospital U.S. Post Officer Drawer 2218 33902	334-5286
Ft. Walton Beach	Poison Control Center Fort Walton Beach Hospital 207 Hospital Drive, North East 32548	243-7611 Ext. 223
Gainesville	Poison Control Center Alachua General Hospital 315 South West 10th Street 32601	372-4321 Ext. 333
	Poison Information Center J. Hillis Miller Health Center University of Florida 32601	392-3591
Jacksonville	Poison Control Center, St. Vincent's Hospital Barrs Street & St. Johns Avenue 32204	389-7751 Ext. 315
Key West	Poison Control Center Monroe General Hospital Stock Island 33040	294-3741 Ext. 237
Lakeland	Poison Control Center, Lakeland General Hospital, Lakeland Hills Boulevard P.O. Box 480 33801	686-1111 Ext. 599 597
Leesburg	Poison Control Center Leesburg General Hospital 600 East Dixie 32748	787-7222 Ext. 221
Melbourne	Poison Control Center, Brevard Hospital 1350 South Hickory Street 32901	727-7000 Ext. 704 741, 798
Miami	Poison Control Center Jackson Memorial Hospital 1700 North West 10th Avenue 33136	371-9611 Ext. 378
Miami Beach	Poison Control Center, Mt. Sinai Hospital 4300 Alton Road 33140	532-3611 Ext. 3333
Naples	Poison Control Center Naples Community Hospital 350 7th Street North 33940	649-3131 Ext. 221
Ocala	Poison Control Center Munroe Memorial Hospital 1410 South Orange Street 32670	629-7911 Ext. 15
Orlando	Poison Control Center Orange Memorial Hospital 1416 South Orange Avenue 32806	241-2411 Ext. 656

Panama City   Poison Control Center   785-7411
Memorial Hospital of Bay County   Ext. 652
600 North MacArthur Avenue 32401

Pensacola   Poison Control Center, Baptist Hospital   434-4811
1000 West Moreno Street 32501   Ext. 518, 519

Plant City   Poison Control Center   752-1188
South Florida Baptist Hospital
Drawer H 33566

Pompano Beach   Poison Control Center   941 8300
North Brovard Hospital   Ext. 710
201 Sample Road 33064

Punta Gorda   Poison Control Center   639-2191
Medical Center Hospital   Ext. 129
809 East Marion Avenue 33950

Rockledge   Poison Control Center   636-2211
Wuesthoff Memorial Hospital   Ext. 506
110 Longwood Avenue 32955   507

St. Petersburg   Poison Control Center   894-1161
Bayfront Medical Center, Inc.   Ext. 241
701 6th Street, South 33701   242

Sarasota   Poison Control Center   955-1111
Sarasota Memorial Hospital   Ext. 1241
1901 Arlington Avenue 33579

Tallahassee   Poison Control Center, Tallahassee   877-2181
Memorial Hospital, North Magnolia Drive &   Ext. 299
Miccosukee Road 32303

Tampa   Poison Control Center   251-6995
Tampa General Hospital
Davis Islands 33606

Titusville   Poison Control Center   269-1100
Jess Parrish Memorial Hospital   Ext. 474
951 North Washington Avenue 32780

W. Palm Beach   Poison Control Center   655-5511
Good Samaritan Hospital   Ext. 341
1300 North Dixie Highway 33402   342, 343

Winter Haven   Poison Control Center   293-1121
Winter Haven Hospital, Inc.   Ext. 222
200 Avenue F, North East 33880

Georgia

State Coordinator
Dept. of Public Health, Atlanta 30334   656-4839

Albany   Poison Information Center   436-5741
Phoebe Putney Memorial Hospital   Ext. 155
417 3rd Avenue, P.O. Box 1151 31705

Athens   Poison Control Center   549-9977
Athens General Hospital   Ext. 223
797 Cobb Street 30601

Atlanta   Poison Control Center   523-4711
Grady Memorial Hospital   Ext. 893
80 Butler Street, South East 30303

Augusta   Poison Information Center   724-7171
University Hospital, University Place 30902   Ext. 233

Columbus   Poison Information Center   324-4711
The Medical Center   Ext. 431
19th Street & 18th Avenue 31902

Macon   Poison Control Center, Macon Hospital   743-4113
777 Hemlock Street 31201   Ext. 314, 315, 309

Rome   Poison Control Center, Floyd Hospital   235-0451
Turner & McCall Boulevard 30161

Savannah   Poison Information Center   345-3200
Memorial Hospital   Ext. 367
Waters Avenue at 63rd Street 31404

Thomasville   Poison Control Center   226-4121
John D. Archbold Memorial Hospital   Ext. 209
900 Gordon Avenue 31792

Valdosta   Poison Control Center   242-3450
Pineview General Hospital   Ext. 249
Pendleton Park 31601   250

Waycross   Poison Control Center, Memorial Hospital   283-3030
410 Darling Avenue 31501   Ext. 240, 241, 242

Guam

State Coordinator
Dept. of Public Health & Social Services 42-4158
Agana 96910

Agana Poison Control Center 746-9171
Guam Memorial Hospital 96910

Hawaii

State Coordinator
Dept. of Health, Honolulu 96801 531-7776

Honolulu Poison Control Center 531-3511
Kauikeolani Children's Hospital
226 North Kuakini Street 96817

Idaho

State Coordinator
State Dept. of Health, Boise 83701 384-2494

Boise Poison Information Center 342-7781
St. Luke's Hospital Pharmacy
130 East Bannock 83702

Illinois

State Coordinator
Dept. of Public Health, Springfield 62706 525-7747

Aurora Poison Control Center 896-4611
Copley Memorial Hospital Ext. 725
Lincoln & Weston Avenues 60507

Poison Control Center, St. Charles Hospital 897-8714
400 East New York Street 60507 Ext. 50

Belleville Poison Control Center, Memorial Hospital 233-7750
4501 North Park Drive 62223 Ext. 250, 251

Belvidere Poison Control Center, Highland Hospital 547-5441
1625 South State Street 61008 Ext. 367

Berwyn Poison Control Center 484-2211
MacNeal Memorial Hospital Ext. 311
3249 Oak Park Avenue 60402 312, 314

Bloomington Poison Control Center, Mennonite Hospital 828-5241
807 North Main 61701 Ext. 311

Poison Control Center, St. Joseph Hospital 829-9481
2200 East Washington 61701 Ext. 352, 354

Cairo Poison Control Center, St. Mary's Hospital 734-2400
2020 Cedar Street 62914 Ext. 42
Night: 45

Canton Poison Control Center 647-5240
Graham Hospital Association Ext. 230
210 West Walnut Street 61520

Carbondale Poison Control Center 457-4101
Doctors Memorial Hospital
404 West Main Street 62901

Carthage Poison Control Center, Memorial Hospital 357-3133
End South Adams Street 62321 Ext. 57

Centralia Poison Control Center, St. Mary's Hospital 532-6731
400 North Pleasant Avenue 62801 Ext. 626
Night: 629

Champaign Poison Control Center 337-2533
Burnham City Hospital
311 East Stoughton Street 61820

Chanute AFB Poison Control Center 495-3133
USAF Hospital, Chanute AFB 61866 495-3134
(Limited for treatment of military personnel and
families, except for indicated civilian emergencies)

Chicago Chicago Master Center 942-5969
Presbyterian-St. Lukes Hospital
1753 West Congress Parkway 60612

Chester Poison Control Center, Memorial Hospital 826-2388
1900 State Street 62233 Ext. 44

Danville Poison Control Center 443-5221
Lake View Memorial Hospital
812 North Logan Avenue 61832

Poison Control Center, St. Elizabeth Hospital 442-6300
600 Sager Avenue 61832

Decatur	Poison Control Center Decatur Memorial Hospital 2300 North Edward Street 62526	877-8121 Ext. 676 675
	Poison Control Center, St. Mary's Hospital 1800 East Lake Shore Drive 62525	429-2966 Ext. 640
Des Plaines	Poison Control Center Holy Family Hospital 100 North River Road 60016	299-2281 Ext. 856
East St. Louis	Poison Control Center Christian Welfare Hospital 1509 Illinois Avenue 62201	874-7076 Ext. 232
	Poison Control Center, St. Mary's Hospital 129 North 8th Street 62201	274-1900 Ext. 204
Effingham	Poison Control Center St. Anthony's Memorial Hospital 503 North Maple 62401	342-2121 Ext. 67
Elgin	Poison Control Center, St. Joseph's Hospital 277 Jefferson Avenue 60120	741-5400 Ext. 65-69
	Poison Control Center, Sherman Hospital 934 Center Street 60120	742-9800 Ext. 682
Elmhurst	Poison Control Center Memorial Hospital of DuPage County 315 Schiller Street 60127	833-1400 Ext. 551 552
Evanston	Poison Control Center, Community Hospital 2040 Brown Avenue 60201	869-5400 Ext. 54 Night: 58
	Poison Control Center, Evanston Hospital 2650 Ridge Avenue 60201	492-6460
	Poison Control Center, St. Francis Hospital 355 Ridge Avenue 60202	492-2440
Evergreen Park	Poison Control Center Little Company of Mary Hospital 2800 West 95th Street 60642	422-6200 HI 5-6000 Ext. 221
Fairbury	Poison Control Center, Fairbury Hospital 519 South 5th Street 61739	692-2346
Freeport	Poison Control Center Freeport Memorial Hospital 420 South Harlem 61032	233-4131 Ext. 228
Galena	Poison Control Center The Galena Hospital District Summit Street 61036	777-1340
Galesburg	Poison Control Center Galesburg Cottage Hospital 674 North Seminary Street 61401	343-4121 Ext. 356
	Poison Control Center, St. Mary's Hospital 239 South Cherry Street 61401	343-3161 Ext. 210
Granite City	Poison Control Center St. Elizabeth Hospital 2100 Madison Avenue 62040	876-2020 Ext. 224
Harvey	Poison Control Center Ingalls Memorial Hospital 15510 Page Avenue 60426	333-2300 Ext. 787 792
Highland	Poison Control Center, St. Joseph Hospital 1515 Main Street 62249	654-2171 Ext. 243
Highland Park	Poison Control Center Highland Park Hospital Foundation 718 Glenview Avenue 60035	432-8000 Ext. 561 562, 563
Hinsdale	Poison Control Center Hinsdale Sanitarium & Hospital 120 North Oak Street 60521	323-2100 Ext. 336
Hoopeston	Poison Control Center Hoopeston Community Memorial Hospital 701 East Orange 60942	283-5531
Jacksonville	Poison Control Center Passavant Memorial Area Hospital 1600 West Walnut Street 62650	245-9541 Ext. 222
Joliet	Poison Control Center, St. Joseph's Hospital 333 North Madison Street 60435	725-7133 Ext. 793
	Poison Control Center, Silver Cross Hospital 600 Walnut Street 60432	727-1711 Ext. 731, 780, 679, 680

Kankakee	Poison Control Center, Riverside Hospital 350 North Wall Street 60901	933-1671 Ext. 606
	Poison Control Center, St. Mary's Hospital 150 South Fifth Avenue 60901	939-4111 Ext. 735
Kewanee	Poison Control Center Kewanee Public Hospital 719 Elliott Street 61443	853-3361 Ext. 219
Lake Forest	Poison Control Center, Lake Forest Hospital 660 Northwestmoreland Road 60045	234-5600 Ext. 608
LaSalle	Poison Control Center, St. Mary's Hospital 1015 O'Conor Avenue 61301	233-0607
Libertyville	Poison Control Center Condell Memorial Hospital Cleveland & Stewart Avenues 60048	362-2900 Ext. 325 326
Lincoln	Poison Control Center Abraham Lincoln Memorial Hospital 315 Eighth Street 62656	732-2161 Ext. 346
McHenry	Poison Control Center, McHenry Hospital 3516 West Waukegan Road 60050	385-2200 Ext. 614
Macomb	Poison Control Center McDonough District Hospital 525 East Grant Street 61455	833-4101
Mattoon	Poison Control Center Memorial Hospital, District of Coles County 2101 Champaign Avenue 61938	234-8881 Ext. 43 Night: 29
Maywood	Poison Control Center Loyola University Hospital 2160 South 1st Avenue 60153	531-3886
Melrose Park	Poison Control Center, Westlake Hospital 1225 Superior Street 60160	681-3000 Ext. 226, 239
Mendota	Poison Control Center Mendota Community Hospital Memorial Drive 61342	7461 Ext. 20
Moline	Poison Control Center Moline Public Hospital 635 10th Avenue 61265	762-3651 Ext. 232
Monmouth	Poison Control Center Community Memorial Hospital West Harlem Avenue 61462	734-3141 Ext. 224
Mt. Carmel	Poison Control Center Wabash General Hospital 1418 College Drive 62863	262-4121 Ext. 231
Mt. Vernon	Poison Control Center Good Samaritan Hospital 605 North 12th Street 62864	242-4600 Ext. 303
Naperville	Poison Control Center, Edward Hospital South Washington Street 60540	355-0450 Ext. 326
Normal	Poison Control Center, Brokaw Hospital Franklin & Virginia Avenues 61761	829-7685 Ext. 274
Oak Lawn	Poison Control Center Christ Community Hospital 4440 West 95th Street 60453	423-7000 Ext. 659, 660 & 661
Oak Park	Poison Control Center West Suburban Hospital 518 North Austin Boulevard 60302	383-6200 Ext. 6747
Olney	Poison Control Center Richland Memorial Hospital 800 East Locust Street 62450	395-2131
Ottawa	Poison Control Center Ryburn Memorial Hospital 701 Clinton Street 61350	433-3100
Park Ridge	Poison Control Center Lutheran General Hospital 1775 Dempster Street 60068	692-2210 Ext. 1220 Night: 1460
Pekin	Poison Control Center Pekin Memorial Hospital 14th & Court 61554	347-1151 Ext. 233 241

Peoria	Poison Control Center, Methodist Hospital 221 North East Glen Oak Avenue 61603	685-6511 Ext. 250
	Poison Control Center Proctor Community Hospital 5409 North Knoxville 61614	691-4702 Ext. 791 792
	Poison Control Center, St. Francis Hospital 530 North East Glen Oak Avenue 61603	674-2943
Peru	Poison Control Center, Peoples Hospital 925 W Street 61354	223-3300 Ext. 55 Night: 40
Pittsfield	Poison Control Center Illini Community Hospital 640 West Washington Street 62363	285-2115 Ext. 238 Night: 213
Princeton	Poison Control Center Perry Memorial Hospital 530 East Park Avenue 61356	875-2811 Ext. 311
Quincy	Poison Control Center, Blessing Hospital 1005 Broadway 62301	223-5811 Ext. 211, 212
	Poison Control Center, St. Mary's Hospital 1415 Vermont Street 62301	223-1200 Ext. 275
Rockford	Poison Control Center Rockford Memorial Hospital 2400 North Rockton Avenue 61103	968-6861 Ext. 441
	Poison Control Center St. Anthony's Hospital 5666 East State Street 61108	226-2041
	Poison Control Center Swedish-American Hospital 1316 Charles Street 61108	968-6898 Ext. 602
Rock Island	Poison Control Center St. Anthony's Hospital 767 30th Street 61202	788-7631 Ext. 771 772
St. Charles	Poison Control Center, Delnor Hospital 975 North Fifth Avenue 60174	584-3300 Ext. 229, 218 Night: 286
Scott AFB	Poison Control Center USAF Medical Center 62225	256-7595
Springfield	Poison Control Center, Memorial Hospital 1st & Miller Streets 62701	528-2041 Ext. 333
	Poison Control Center, St. John's Hospital 701 East Mason Street 62701	544-6451 Ext. 375
Streator	Poison Control Center, St. Mary's Hospital 111 East Spring Street 61364	672-3189 Ext. 221
Urbana	Poison Control Center Carle Foundation Hospital 611 West Park Street 61801	337-3313
	Poison Control Center, Mercy Hospital 1400 West Park Avenue 61801	337-2131
Waukegan	Poison Control Center, St. Therese Hospital West Waukegan Street 60085	688-6470 688-6471
	Poison Control Center Victory Memorial Hospital 1324 North Sheridan Road 60085	688-4181
Woodstock	Poison Control Center Memorial Hospital for McHenry County 527 West South Street 60098	338-2500 Ext. 32
Zion	Poison Control Center, Zion-Benton Hospital 2500 Emmaus Avenue 60099	872-4561 Ext. 240

Indiana

	State Coordinator State Board of Health, Indianapolis 46206	633-5490
Anderson	Poison Control Center St. John's Hickey Memorial Hospital 2015 Jackson Street 46014	694-2511 Ext. 251
Angola	Poison Control Center Cameron Memorial Hospital, Inc. 416 East Maumee Street 46703	665-2141 Ext. 42 665-2166
East Chicago	Poison Control Center, St. Catherine Hospital 4321 Fir Street 46312	EX 7-3080

Elkhart	Poison Control Center Elkhart General Hospital 600 East Boulevard 46514	523-5350 Ext. 215
Evansville	Poison Control Center, Deaconess Hospital 600 Mary Street 47710	426-3405
	Poison Control Center, St. Mary's Hospital 3700 Washington Avenue 47715	477-6261
	Poison Control Center Welborn Memorial Baptist Hospital 412 South East 4th Street 47713	423-3103 Ext. 336 Night: 253
Fort Wayne	Poison Control Center Parkview Memorial Hospital 220 Randalia Drive 46805	484-6636 Ext. 530
	Poison Control Center, St. Joseph's Hospital 700 Broadway 46802	742-4121 Ext. 211
Frankfort	Poison Control Center Clinton County Hospital 1300 South Jackson Street 46041	654-4451
Gary	Poison Control Center Methodist Hospital of Gary, Inc. 600 Grant Street 46402	882-9461 Ext. 709
Goshen	Poison Control Center Goshen General Hospital 200 High Park Avenue 46526	533-2141 Ext. 462
Hammond	Poison Control Center St. Margaret Hospital 25 Douglas Street 46320	WE 2-2300 Ext. 700
Indianapolis	Poison Control Center Marion County General Hospital 960 Locke Street 46202	630-7351
	Poison Control Center Methodist Hospital of Indiana, Inc. 1604 North Capitol Avenue 46202	924-8355
Kokomo	Poison Control Center Howard Community Hospital 3500 South La Fountain Street 46901	453-0702 Ext. 218
Lafayette	Poison Control Center, Purdue University Student Health Center 47907	749-2441 Ext. 245
	Poison Control Center, St. Elizabeth Hospital 1501 Hartford Street 47904	742-0221 Ext. 428, 421
La Grange	Poison Control Center La Grange County Hospital Route 1 46761	463-2144 Ext. 34
Lebanon	Poison Control Center Witham Memorial Hospital 1124 North Lebanon Street 46052	482-2700 Ext. 44
Madison	Poison Control Center King's Daughters' Hospital 112 Presbyterian Avenue P.O. Box 447 47250	265-5211 Ext. 14
Marion	Poison Control Center Marion General Hospital Wabash & Euclid Avenue 46952	662-1441 Ext. 294 295
Mishawaka	Poison Control Center, St. Joseph Hospital 215 West 4th Street 46544	259-2431
Muncie	Poison Control Center Ball Memorial Hospital 2401 University Avenue 47303	284-3371 Ext. 241 242, 371
Portland	Poison Control Center, Jay County Hospital 505 West Arch Street 47371	726-7131 Ext. 159
Richmond	Poison Control Center Reid Memorial Hospital 1401 Chester Boulevard 47374	962-4545 Ext. 222, 333
Shelbyville	Poison Control Center William S. Major Hospital 150 West Washington Street 46176	392-3211 Ext. 52
South Bend	Poison Control Center Memorial Hospital of South Bend 615 Michigan Street 46601	234-9041 Ext. 258 259
	Poison Control Center, St. Joseph's Hospital 811 East Madison Street 46622	234-2151 Ext. 264

Terre Haute — Poison Control Center, Union Hospital, Inc.
1606 North 7th Street 47804
232-0361
Ext. 229

Iowa

State Coordinator
Department of Health, Des Moines 50319 — 281-5787

Des Moines — Poison Information Center
Raymond Blank Memorial Hospital
1200 Pleasant Street 50308
283-6254

Fort Dodge — Poison Information Center
Bethesda General Hospital
Lutheran Park Road 50501
573-3101
Ext. 230

Iowa City — Poison Information Center
University Hospital
Pharmacy Department 52241
356-1616

Kansas

State Coordinator
State Department of Health, Topeka 66612 — 296-3708

Atchison — Poison Control Center, Atchison Hospital
1301 North 2nd Street 66002
EM 7-2131
Ext. 28

Dodge City — Poison Control Center, Trinity Hospital
1107 6th Street 67801
227-8133

Emporia — Poison Control Center
Newman Memorial Hospital
12th & Chestnut Streets 66801
342-7120
Ext. 330

Fort Scott — Poison Control Center, Mercy Hospital
821 Burke Street 66701
BA 3-2200
Ext. 52

Great Bend — Poison Control Center
Central Kansas Medical Center
3515 Broadway 67530
792-2511
Ext. 115

Hays — Poison Control Center
Hadley Memorial Hospital
201 East 7th Street 67601
625-3441

Kansas City — Poison Control Center, University of Kansas
Medical Center, Dept. of Pharmacology
Rainbow Boulevard at 39th Street 66103
AD 6-5252
Ext. 555

Lawrence — Poison Control Center
Lawrence Memorial Hospital
325 Main Street 66044
843-3680
Ext. 362

Parsons — Poison Control Center
Labette County Medical Center
South 21st Street 67357
421-4880
Ext. 245

Salina — Poison Control Center, St. John's Hospital
139 North Penn Street 67401
TA 7-5591
Ext. 125

Topeka — Poison Control Center
Stormont-Vail Hospital
10th & Washburn Streets 66604
234-9961
Ext. 150

Poison Information Center
State Dept. of Health, State Office Building
Topeka Avenue at 10th 66612
296-3708

Wichita — Poison Control Center
Wesley Hospital, Medical Library
550 North Hillside Avenue 67214
685-2151
Ext. 377

Kentucky

State Coordinator
State Department of Health
Frankfort 40601
564-4830

Ashland — Poison Control Center
King's Daughters' Hospital
2201 Lexington Avenue 41101
325-7755
Ext. 291

Fort Thomas — Poison Control Center, St. Luke Hospital
85 North Grand Avenue 41075
441-6100
Ext. 215, 216

Lexington — Poison Control Center
Central Baptist Hospital
1740 South Limestone Street 40503
278-3411
Ext. 152
153

Poison Information Center
University of Kentucky
Medical Center 40506
233-5853

Owensboro	Poison Control Center Owensboro-Daviess County Hospital 811 Hospital Court 42301	683-3513 Ext. 275
Paducah	Poison Control Center Western Baptist Hospital 2501 Kentucky Avenue 42001	444-6361 Ext. 221

Louisiana

	State Coordinator State Department of Health New Orleans 70160	527-5822
Bogalusa	Poison Information Center Washington-St. Tammany Charity Hospital 400 Memphis Street 70427	735-1322
Monroe	Poison Control Center, St. Francis Hospital 309 Jackson Street 71201	325-6454
New Orleans	Louisiana Poison Control Center of New Orleans U.S. Public Health Service Hospital 210 State Street 70118	899-3409
Shreveport	Poison Control Center T. E. Schumpert Memorial Hospital 915 Margaret Place 71101	422-0709 424-6411 Ext. 240, 271

Maine

	State Coordinator Dept. of Health & Welfare, Augusta 04330	623-4511
Togus	Poison Control Center Veterans Administration Center Kennebec County 04330	623-8411 Ext. 283 305

Maryland

	State Coordinator State Department of Health Baltimore 21201	382-2668
Annapolis	Poison Control Center Anne Arundel General Hospital Franklin & Cathedral Streets 21401	268-4444 Ext. 277
Baltimore	Poison Information Center Baltimore City Hospital 4940 Eastern Avenue 21224	DI 2-0800
	Poison Control Center Johns Hopkins Hospital 601 North Broadway 21205	955-6371
	Poison Control Center University of Maryland Hospital Redwood & Greene Streets 21201	955-7592 Night: 955-8761
Bethesda	Poison Control Center Suburban Hospital Emergency Room 8600 Old Georgetown Road 20014	530-3880
Cumberland	Tri-State Poison Control Center Sacred Heart Hospital 900 Seton Drive 21401	729-5200
Easton	Poison Control Center, Memorial Hospital South Washington Street 21601	822-5555
Hagerstown	Poison Control Center Washington County Hospital King & Antietam Streets 21740	733-3000
Silver Spring	Poison Control Center, Holy Cross Hospital Forest Glen Road 20910	495-1225

Massachusetts

	State Coordinator State Dept. of Public Health, Boston 02133	727-2700
Boston	Poison Information Center Childrens Medical Center 300 Longwood Avenue 02115	232-2120
Fall River	Poison Control Center, Union Hospital 300 Hanover Street 02720	679-6405 Ext. 232
New Bedford	Poison Control Center, St. Luke's Hospital 52 Brigham Street 02740	997-1515 Ext. 311

Springfield	Poison Control Center, Mercy Hospital 233 Carew Street 01104	788-7321 Ext. 229
	Poison Control Center Springfield Hospital Medical Center 759 Chestnut Street 01107	787-3200 Ext. 3233
	Poison Control Center Wesson Memorial Hospital 140 High Street 01105	ST 5-1241 Ext. 218
Worcester	Poison Information Center Worcester City Hospital 26 Queen Street 01610	799-7094

Michigan

	State Coordinator Department of Public Health Lansing 48914	373-1320
Adrian	Poison Control Center Emma L. Bixby Hospital 818 Riverside Avenue 49221	265-6161
Ann Arbor	Poison Control Center University of Michigan Medical Center 48104	764-5102
Battle Creek	Poison Control Center, Community Hospital 200 Tomkins Street 49016	WO 3-5521
Bay City	Poison Control Center, Mercy Hospital 100 15th Street 48706	TW 5-8511
Berrien Center	Poison Control Center Berrien General Hospital Dean's Hill Road 49102	471-7761
Coldwater	Poison Control Center Community Health Center of Branch County 274 East Chicago Street 49036	279-9501
Detroit	Poison Control Center, Children's Hospital 5224 St. Antoine Street 48202	833-1000
	Poison Information Center City Health Department 1151 Taylor Avenue 48202	TR 2-1540
	Poison Control Center Mount Carmel Mercy Hospital 6071 West Outer Drive 48235	864-5400
Eloise	Poison Control Center Wayne County General Hospital 30712 Michigan Avenue 48132	722-2500 Ext. 6230 6231
Flint	Poison Control Center, Hurley Hospital 6th Avenue & Begole 48502	CE 2-1161
Grand Rapids	Poison Control Center Blodgett Memorial Hospital 1840 Wealthy, South East 49506	456-5301
	Poison Control Center, Butterworth Hospital 100 Michigan, North East 49503	451-3591
	Poison Control Center Grand Rapids Osteopathic Hospital 1919 Boston Street, South East 49506	452-5151
	Poison Control Center, St. Mary's Hospital 201 Lafayette, South East 49503	459-3131
Hancock	Poison Control Center, St. Joseph's Hospital 200 Michigan Avenue 49930	482-1122
Kalamazoo	Poison Control Center Bronson Methodist Hospital 252 East Lovell Street 49006	342-9821
Lansing	Poison Control Center St. Lawrence Hospital 1210 West Saginaw Street 48914	372-3610
Marquette	Poison Control Center, St. Luke's Hospital West College Avenue 49855	CAnal 6-3551
Midland	Poison Control Center, Midland Hospital 4005 Orchard Drive 48640	TE 5-6711
Monroe	Poison Control Center Memorial Hospital of Monroe 700 Stewart Road 48161	CH 1-6500

Petoskey Poison Control Center Diamond
Little Traverse Hospital 7-2551
416 Connable 49770

Pontiac Poison Control Center 338-9111
St. Joseph Mercy Hospital
900 Woodward Avenue 48053

Port Huron Poison Control Center, Mercy Hospital Yukon
2601 Electric Avenue 48060 5-9531

Saginaw Poison Control Center 753-3411
Saginaw General Hospital
1447 North Harrison Road 48602

Traverse City Poison Control Center 947-6140
Munson Medical Center
Traverse City 49684

Minnesota

State Coordinator
State Department of Health 378-1150
Minneapolis 55440

Bemidji Poison Information Center 751-5430
Bemidji Hospital 56601 Ext. 40

Brainerd Poison Information Center 829-2861
St. Joseph's Hospital 56401

Crookston Poison Information Center 281-4682
Riverview Hospital 56716 Ext. 250

Duluth Poison Information Center 727-6636
St. Luke's Hospital 55805 Ext. 211

Poison Information Center 727-4551
St. Mary's Hospital Ext. 359
407 East 3rd Street 55805 Night: 291

Fergus Falls Poison Information Center 736-5475
Lake Region Hospital 56537 Ext. 222

Fridley Poison Information Center, Unity Hospital 786-2200
550 Osborne Road 55432 Ext. 221, 222, 223

Mankato Poison Information Center 387-1851
Immanuel-St. Joseph's Hospital
325 Garden Boulevard 56001

Marshall Poison Information Center 532-2263
Louis Weiner Memorial Hospital 56258 Sta. 31

Minneapolis Fairview Hospital 332-0282
2312 South 6th Street 55406 Ext. 313

Hennepin County General Hospital 330-3930
620 South 6th Street 55415

Poison Information Center 378-1150
Minnesota Dept. of Health Ext. 352
717 Delaware Street South East 55440 Night: 929-
6491, 784-1869

North Memorial Hospital 588-0616
3220 Lowry Avenue North 55422 Ext. 342

Northwestern Hospital 332-7266
810 East 27th Street 55407

Morris Poison Information Center 589-1313
Stevens County Memorial Hospital 56267 Sta. 1

Rochester Poison Information Center 282-4461
Rochester Methodist Hospital 55901 Ext. 5250

St. Cloud Poison Information Center 251-2700
St. Cloud Hospital 56301 Ext. 151, 152
Night: 221

St. Paul Poison Information Center 227-8611
Bethesda Lutheran Hospital Ext. 301
559 Capitol Boulevard 55101

Children's Hospital 227-6521
311 Pleasant Avenue 55102 Ext. 343

St. John's Hospital, 403 Maria Avenue 55106 228-3132

St. Joseph's Hospital 222-2861
69 West Exchange 55102 Ext. 348, 349

St. Luke's Hospital, 300 Pleasant Avenue 228-8201
c/o Emergency Room 55102

	Poison Information Center St. Paul-Ramsey Hospital 640 Jackson Street 55101	222-4260 Ext. 215
Virginia	Poison Information Center Virginia Municipal Hospital 55792	741-3340
Willmar	Poison Information Center Rice Memorial Hospital 56201	235-4543 Ext. 56
Worthington	Poison Information Center Worthington Municipal Hospital 56187	376-4141 Ext. 32 Night: 376-6834

Mississippi

	State Coordinator State Board of Health, Jackson 39205	354-6650
Brandon	Poison Control Center Rankin General Hospital 350 Grossgates Boulevard 39042	825-2811 Ext. 626
Columbia	Poison Control Center Marion County General Hospital 39429	736-6303 Ext. 217
Greenwood	Poison Control Center Greenwood-LeFlore Hospital River Road 38930	453-9751 Ext. 231
Hattiesburg	Poison Control Information Center Forrest County General Hospital 400 South 28th Avenue 39401	582-8361 Ext. 46
Jackson	Poison Control Center, Baptist Hospital 1190 North State Street 39201	948-5211 Ext. 201 202, 203
	Poison Control Center St. Dominic-Jackson Memorial Hospital 969 Lakeland Drive 39216	266-5281
	State Board of Health Division of Preventable Disease Control 39205	354-6650
Keesler AFB (Biloxi)	Poison Control Center USAF Hospital Keesler Keesler Air Force Base 39534	432-1521 Ext. 284
Laurel	Poison Control Center Jones County Community Hospital Jefferson Street at 13th Avenue 39440	425-1441 Ext. 20, 48
Meridian	Poison Control Center, St. Joseph Hospital Highway 39, North 39301	483-6211 Ext. 54, 42
Pascagoula	Poison Control Center Singing River Hospital Highway 90E 39567	762-6121 Ext. 761
University	Poison Control Center, School of Pharmacy University of Mississippi 38677	234-1522
Vicksburg	Poison Control Center Mercy Hospital-Street Memorial 100 McAuley Drive 39181	636-2121 Ext. 302 255, 256

Missouri

	State Coordinator Missouri Division of Health Jefferson City 65101	635-4111
Cape Girardeau	Poison Control Center, St. Francis Hospital 825 Good Hope Street 63701	334-4461 Ext. 49
Columbia	Poison Control Center University of Missouri Medical Center 807 Stadium Boulevard 65201	442-5111
Hannibal	Poison Control Center St. Elizabeth Hospital 109 Virginia Street 63401	221-0414 Ext. 213
Joplin	Poison Control Center, St. John's Hospital 2727 McClelland Boulevard 64801	781-2727 Ext. 276
Kansas City	Poison Control Center Children's Mercy Hospital 24th & Gillham Road 64108	471-0626 Ext. 220
	Poison Control Center, Kansas City General Hospital and Medical Center 23rd & Cherry Streets 64108	HA 1-8060 Ext. 257 235

Kirksville	Poison Control Center Kirksville Osteopathic Hospital 800 West Jefferson Street 63501	665-4611 Ext. 240
Poplar Bluff	Poison Control Center, Lucy Lee Hospital 330 North 2nd Street 63901	785-7721 Ext. 33
Rolla	Poison Control Center Phelps County Memorial Hospital 1000 West 10th Street 65401	364-3100 Ext. 31
St. Joseph	Poison Control Center Methodist Hospital and Medical Center 8th & Faraon Streets 64501	232-8461 Ext. 277
St. Louis	Poison Control Center, Cardinal Glennon Children's Memorial Hospital 1465 South Grand Avenue 63104	865-4000 Ext. 417
	Poison Control Center St. Louis Children's Hospital 500 South Kingshighway 63110	367-6880 Ext. 220
Springfield	Poison Control Center Lester E. Cox Medical Center 1423 North Jefferson Street 65802	865-9631 Ext. 253 254
	Poison Control Center, St. John's Hospital 1235 East Cherokee 65804	881-88.. Ext. 248, 241
West Plains	Poison Control Center West Plains Memorial Hospital 1103 Alaska Avenue 65775	256-3141 Ext. 8

Montana

	State Coordinator State Department of Health, Helena 59601	449-2544
Bozeman	Poison Control Center Bozeman Deaconess Hospital 15 West Lamme 59715	586-5431
Helena	Poison Control Center St. Peter's Hospital 59601	442-2480 Ext. 317

Nebraska

	State Coordinator State Department of Health, Lincoln 68509	477-5211
Lincoln	Poison Control Center Bryan Memorial Hospital 4848 Sumner Street 68506	473-3244
Omaha	Poison Control Center Children's Memorial Hospital 44th & Dewey Streets 68105	553-5400 Poison Control

Nevada

	State Coordinator Dept. of Health & Welfare Carson City 89701	882-7458
Las Vegas	Poison Control Center Southern Nevada Memorial Hospital 1800 West Charleston Boulevard 89102	385-1277
Reno	Poison Control Center Washoe Medical Center Kirman & Mills Streets 89502	785-4129

New Hampshire

	State Coordinator Dept. of Health & Welfare Concord 03301	225-6611
Hanover	Poison Information Center Mary Hitchcock Hospital 2 Maynard Street 03755	643-4000

New Jersey

	State Coordinator State Dept. of Health, Trenton 08625	292-5616
Atlantic City	Poison Control Center, Atlantic City Hospital 1925 Pacific Avenue 08401	344-4081 Ext. 228
Belleville	Poison Control Center, Clara Maass Hospital 1A Franklin Avenue 07109	751-1000 Ext. 781

Boonton	Poison Control Center, Riverside Hospital Powerville Road 07005	334-5000 Ext. 55
Bridgeton	Poison Control Center, Bridgeton Hospital Irving Avenue 08302	451-6600
Camden	Poison Control Center, West Jersey Hospital Mt. Ephraim & Atlantic Avenues 08104	963-8830 Ext. 351
Denville	Poison Control Center, St. Clare's Hospital Pocono Road 07834	627-3000 Ext. 208
East Orange	Poison Control Center East Orange General Hospital 300 Central Avenue 07019	672-8400 Ext. 223
Elizabeth	Poison Control Center St. Elizabeth Hospital 225 Williamson Street 07207	289-4000 Ext. 351
Englewood	Poison Control Center, Englewood Hospital 350 Engle Avenue 07631	568-3400 Ext. 391
Flemington	Poison Control Center Hunterdon Medical Center Route 31 08822	782-2121
Hasbrouck Heights	Poison Control Center Hasbrouck Heights Hospital 214 Terrace Avenue 07604	288-0800
Livingston	Poison Control Center St. Barnabas Medical Center Old Short Hills Road 07039	992-5500 Ext. 467
Long Branch	Poison Control Center Monmouth Medical Center 255 2nd Avenue 07740	222-2210
Montclair	Poison Control Center Mountainside Hospital Bay & Highland Avenues 07042	746-6000 Ext. 234
Morristown	Poison Control Center, All Souls Hospital 95 Mount Kemble Avenue 07960	538-0900 Ext. 220
Mount Holly	Poison Control Center Burlington County Memorial Hospital 175 Madison Avenue 08060	267-0700 Ext. 255
Neptune	Poison Control Center Jersey Shore Medical Center-Fitkin 1945 Corlies Avenue 07753	988-1818
Newark	Poison Control Center Children's Hospital of Newark United Hospitals 15 South 9th Street 07107	484-8000 Ext. 419
	Poison Control Center Newark Beth Israel Hospital 201 Lyons Avenue 07112	923-6000
New Brunswick	Poison Control Center Middlesex General Hospital 180 Somerset Street 08901	828-3000
	Poison Control Center St. Peter's General Hospital Easton Avenue 08903	545-8000 Ext. 329
Newton	Poison Control Center Newton Memorial Hospital 175 High Street 07860	383-2121 Ext. 226
Orange	Poison Control Center Hospital Center at Orange 188 South Essex Avenue 07051	678-1100 Ext. 231
Passaic	Poison Control Center, St. Mary's Hospital 211 Pennington Avenue 07055	473-1000 Ext. 341
Paterson	Poison Control Center Paterson General Hospital 528 Market Street 07501	684-6900 Ext. 330
Perth Amboy	Poison Control Center Perth Amboy General Hospital 530 New Brunswick Avenue 08861	442-3700 Ext. 374
Phillipsburg	Poison Control Center, Warren Hospital 185 Roseberry Street 08865	859-1500 Ext. 278
Point Pleasant	Poison Control Center Point Pleasant Hospital Osborn Avenue & River Front 08743	892-1100 Ext. 266

Princeton	Poison Control Center, Princeton Hospital 253 Witherspoon Street 08540	921-7700 Ext. 241
Saddle Brook	Poison Control Center Saddle Brook Hospital 300 Market Street 07662	843-6700
Somers Point	Poison Control Center Shore Memorial Hospital New York & Sunny Avenues 08244	927-3501 Ext. 208
Somerville	Poison Control Center, Somerset Hospital Rehill Avenue 08876	725-4000 Ext. 203
Summit	Poison Control Center, Overlook Hospital 193 Morris Avenue 07901	273-8100 Ext. 417
Teaneck	Poison Control Center, Holy Name Hospital 718 Teaneck Road 07666	837-3070 Ext. 355
Trenton	Poison Control Center, Helene Fuld Hospital 750 Brunswick Avenue 08638	396-6575 Ext. 378
Union	Poison Control Center Memorial General Hospital 100 Galloping Hill Road 07083	687-1900 Ext. 238

New Mexico

	State Coordinator Department of Public Health Santa Fe 87501	827-2663
Alamogordo	Poison Control Center Gerald Champion Memorial Hospital 1209 9th Street 88310	437-3770 Ext. 260
Albuquerque	Poison Control Center Bernalillo County Indian Hospital 2211 Lomas Boulevard, North East 87106	265-4411
Carlsbad	Poison Control Center Carlsbad Regional Medical Center Northgate Unit, Box 1479 88220	887-3521 Ext. 266
Clovis	Poison Control Center Clovis Memorial Hospital Box 231, 1210 Thornton Street 88101	763-4493 Ext. 131
Las Cruces	Poison Control Center Memorial General Hospital Alameda & Lohman 88001	524-8641 Ext. 25, 61
Raton	Poison Control Center Miners' Hospital of New Mexico South 6th Street 87740	445-2741 Ext. 26
Roswell	Poison Control Center Eastern New Mexico Medical Center 405 Country Club Road 88201	622-8170 Ext. 26

New York

	State Coordinator State Department of Health, Albany 12208	RG 4-2121
Albany	Poison Control Center Albany Medical Center New Scotland Avenue 12208	462-7521
Binghamton	Poison Control Center Binghamton General Hospital Mitchell Avenue 13903	772-1100 Ext. 431
	Poison Control Center Our Lady of Lourdes Memorial Hospital 169 Riverside Drive 13904	729-6521
Buffalo	Poison Control Center Buffalo Children's Hospital 219 Bryant Street 14222	878-7374 878-7503
Dunkirk	Poison Control Center Brooks Memorial Hospital 10 West 6th Street 14048	366-1111 Ext. 414 415
East Meadow	Poison Control Center Meadowbrook Hospital P.O. Box 175 11554	542-2323 542-2324
Elmira	Poison Control Center Arnot Ogden Memorial Hospital Roe Avenue & Grove Street 14901	734-5221 Ext. 237 238, 331
	Poison Control Center, St. Joseph's Hospital 555 East Market Street 14901	733-6541 Ext. 213, 271

Endicott	Poison Control Center Ideal Hospital of Endicott 600 High Avenue 13760	754-7171 Ext. 66
Ithaca	Poison Control Center Tompkins County Hospital 1285 Trumansburg Road 14850	272-7480 Ext. 275 283
Jamestown	Poison Control Center Jamestown General Hospital Hospital Park 14701	484-1161 Ext. 52
	Poison Control Center, W. C. A. Hospital 207 Foote Avenue 14701	487-0141
Johnson City	Poison Control Center Wilson Memorial Hospital 33-57 Harrison Street 13790	797-1211 Ext. 268
Kingston	Poison Control Center, Kingston Hospital 396 Broadway 12401	331-3131 Ext. 250
New York	Poison Control Center New York City Department of Health 455 1st Avenue 10016	340-4494
Niagara Falls	Poison Control Center Niagara Falls Memorial Hospital 621 10th Street 14302	285-2571 Ext. 253
Nyack	Poison Control Center, Nyack Hospital North Midland Avenue 10960	EL 8-6200 Ext. 223
Oswego	Poison Control Center, Oswego Hospital 110 West 6th Street 13126	FI 3-1920
Rochester	Poison Control Center University of Rochester Medical Center and Strong Memorial Hospital 260 Crittenden Boulevard 14620	275-3232
Syracuse	Poison Control Center Upstate Medical Center 750 East Adams Street 13210	GR 6-3166
Warsaw	Poison Control Center Wyoming County Community Hospital 400 North Main Street 14569	796-2233
Watertown	Poison Information Center House of the Good Samaritan Hospital Washington & Pratt Streets 13602	782-8110

North Carolina

	State Coordinator State Board of Health, Raleigh 27602	829-3446
Asheville	Poison Control Center Memorial Mission Hospital 509 Biltmore Avenue 28207	252-5331 Ext. 262
Charlotte	Poison Control Center, Mercy Hospital 2000 East 5th Street 28204	334-6831
Durham	Poison Control Center Duke University Hospital Box 3024 27706	684-8111 Ext. 3957
Hendersonville	Poison Control Center Margaret R. Pardee Hospital Fleming Street 28739	693-6522 Ext. 242
Jacksonville	Poison Control Center Onslow Memorial Hospital College Street 28540	347-1241
Wilmington	Poison Control Center New Hanover Memorial Hospital 2431 South 17th Street 28401	763-9021 Ext. 311 312

North Dakota

	State Coordinator State Department of Health Bismarck 58501	224-2348
Bismarck	Poison Control Center Quain and Ranstad Clinic Burleigh County 58501	223-1420 Night: 223-5000 Night: 223-4700
Dickinson	Poison Control Center, St. Joseph's Hospital 7th Street West 58601	225-6771 Ext. 329, 259
Fargo	Poison Control Center North Dakota State University Pharmacology Department 58102	237-8115

North Dakota—Continued

Grand Forks	Poison Control Center Grand Forks Deaconess Hospital 212 South 4th Street, P.O. Box 1718 58201	775-4241
Jamestown	Poison Control Center, Jamestown Hospital 419 5th Street North East 58401	252-1050
Minot	Poison Control Center, St. Joseph's Hospital 304 4th Street 58701	838-0341 Ext. 253
Williston	Poison Control Center, Mercy Hospital Washington Avenue & Broadway 58801	572-2188

Ohio

	State Coordinator Department of Health, Columbus 43216	469-2544
Akron	Poison Control Center, Children's Hospital 182 Bowery Street 44308	253-5531 Ext. 246
Canton	Poison Information Center Aultman Hospital 2600 6th Street, South West 44710	452-9911 Ext. 203 454-5222
Cincinnati	Poison Control Center The Children's Hospital Elland & Bethesda Avenues 45229	281-6161
Cleveland	Poison Control Center Cleveland Academy of Medicine 10525 Carnegie Avenue 44106	231-3500 231-4455
Columbus	Poison Control Center The Children's Hospital 17th Street at Livingston Park 43205	258-9783
Dayton	Poison Control Center U.S. Air Force Hospital Wright-Patterson AFB 45433	257-2968
Mansfield	Poison Control Center Mansfield General Hospital 335 Glessner Avenue 44903	522-3411
Springfield	Poison Control Center, The Community Hospital of Springfield & Clark County 2615 East High Street 45501	323-5531
Toledo	Poison Information Center Maumee Valley Hospital 2025 Arlington Avenue 43609	382-3435
Youngstown	Poison Control Center St. Elizabeth Hospital 1044 Belmont Avenue 44505	746-7231 Ext. 200 201, 204

Oklahoma

	State Coordinator State Department of Health Oklahoma City 73111	427-6232
Lawton	Poison Control Center, Comanche County Memorial Hospital Gore Boulevard 73501	355-8620 Ext. 232 234
Oklahoma City	Poison Control Center State Department of Health Laboratory Services and Communicable Disease Control 3400 North Eastern 73111	427-6232
Ponca City	Poison Control Center, Ponca City Hospital 14th & Virginia Avenue 74601	765-3321 Ext. 372
Tulsa	Poison Control Center Hillcrest Medical Center 1120 South Utica Avenue 74104	584-1351 Ext. 598

Oregon

Portland	Poison Control Registry Pediatrics Department University of Oregon Medical School 3181 South West Sam Jackson Park Road 97201	228-9181 Ext. 370 Night Emergency Room

Pennsylvania

	State Coordinator State Department of Health Harrisburg 17120	787-6436

Allentown	Poison Control Center Allentown Hospital Association 17th & Chew Streets 18102	434-7161 Ext. 226
Chambersburg	Poison Control Center The Chambersburg Hospital 7th & King Streets 17201	264-5171
Chester	Poison Control Center Sacred Heart General Hospital 9th & Wilson Streets 19013	494-0721
Danville	Poison Control Center, George F. Giesinger Memorial Hospital, Montour County 17821	275-1000 Ext. 591
Easton	Poison Control Center, Easton Hospital 21st & Lehigh Streets 18042	258-6221 Ext. 235 210, 321
East Stroudsburg	Poison Control Center General Hospital of Monroe County 206 East Brown Street 18301	421-4000 Ext. 740
Erie	Poison Control Center Erie Osteopathic Hospital 5515 Peach Street 16509	864-4031 Ext. 27
	Poison Control Center Hamot Hospital Association Second & State Streets 16512	455-6711 Ext. 521
	Poison Control Center, St. Vincent Hospital 232 West 25th Street 16512	453-6911 Ext. 216, 345
Hanover	Poison Control Center Hanover General Hospital 300 Highland Avenue 17331	637-3711 Ext. 111
Harrisburg	Poison Control Center, Harrisburg Hospital Front & Mulberry Streets 17101	782-3639
	Poison Control Center, Polyclinic Hospital 3rd and Polyclinic Avenue 17105	782-4141 Ext. 4132
Johnstown	Poison Control Center, Mercy Hospital 1020 Franklin Street 15905	535-5353
Lancaster	Poison Control Center, St. Joseph's Hospital 250 College Avenue 17604	397-2821 Ext. 201
Latrobe	Poison Control Center Latrobe Area Hospital Association 2nd Avenue 15650	539-9711
Lewistown	Poison Control Center, Lewistown Hospital Highland Avenue 17044	248-5411 Ext. 247
Philadelphia	Poison Information Center Department of Public Health University Avenue & Curie Street 19104	WA 2-5523
Pittsburgh	Poison Control Center, Children's Hospital 125 Desoto Street 15213	681-6669
	Poison Control Center St. John's General Hospital 3339 McClure Avenue 15212	766-8300
Scranton	Poison Control Center Community Medical Center 316 Colfax Avenue 18510	343-5566
Sharon	Poison Control Center Sharon General Hospital 740 East State Street 16146	981-1700 Ext. 281
Wilkes-Barre	Poison Control Center The Mercy Hospital of Wilkes-Barre 196 Hanover Street 18703	822-8101 Ext. 274 305, 306
	Poison Control Center Wilkes-Barre General Hospital North River & Auburn Streets 18702	823-1121 Ext. 222
York	Poison Control Center Memorial Osteopathic Hospital 325 South Belmont Street 17403	843-8623 Ext. 274 275
	Poison Control Center, York Hospital George Street & Rathton Road 17403	854-1511

Puerto Rico

	State Coordinator University of Puerto Rico, Rio Piedras	765-4880 765-0615

Aguadilla	Poison Control Center District Hospital of Aguadilla 00603	891-0200
Arecibo	Poison Control Center District Hospital of Arecibo 00613	878-3535
Fajardo	Poison Control Center District Hospital of Fajardo 00649	863-0505
Mayaguez	Poison Control Center Mayaguez Medical Center Department of Health, P.O. Box 1868 00709	832-8686
Ponce	Poison Control Center District Hospital of Ponce 00731	842-8364 842-2080
San Juan	Poison Control Center Medical Center of Puerto Rico	764-3515

Rhode Island

	State Coordinator State Department of Health Providence 02903	521-7100
Kingston	Poison Control Center, College of Pharmacy University of Rhode Island 02881	792-2763
Pawtucket	Poison Control Center, Memorial Hospital Prospect Street 02860	724-1230
Providence	Poison Control Center Rhode Island Hospital 593 Eddy Street 02902	277-4000
	Poison Control Center Roger Williams General Hospital 825 Chalkstone Avenue 02908	521-5055 Ext. 461

South Carolina

	State Coordinator State Board of Health, Columbia 29201	758-5664
Charleston	Poison Control Center Medical College Hospital 80 Barre Street 29401	792-0211 (Ask to page control center)
Columbia	Poison Control Center, Columbia Hospital 2020 Hampton Street 29204	254-7382

South Dakota

	State Coordinator State Department of Health, Pierre 57501	224-5911
Sioux Falls	Poison Control Center, McKennan Hospital 800 East 21st Street 57101	336-3894
Vermillion	Poison Control Center University of South Dakota Department of Pharmacology 57069	624-3432

Tennessee

	State Coordinator State Department of Public Health Nashville 37219	741-3644
Chattanooga	Poison Control Center T. C. Thompson Children's Hospital 1001 Glenwood Drive 37406	624-5020
Columbia	Poison Control Center Maury County Hospital Mt. Pleasant Pike 38401	388-2320 Ext. 49
Jackson	Poison Control Center Madison General Hospital 708 West Forest 38301	424-0424 Ext. 241
Johnson City	Poison Control Center, Memorial Hospital Boone & Fairview Avenue 37601	926-1131 Ext. 330
Knoxville	Poison Control Center University of Tennessee Memorial Research Center Alcoa Highway 37920	971-3261
Memphis	Poison Control Center Le Bonheur Children's Hospital Adams Avenue at Dunlap 38103	525-6541 Ext. 281
Nashville	Poison Control Center, Vanderbilt Hospital 1161 21st Avenue South 37203	322-2351

Texas

<table>
<tr><td></td><td>State Coordinator
State Department of Health, Austin 78756</td><td>GL 3-6631</td></tr>
<tr><td>Abilene</td><td>Poison Control Center
Hendrick Memorial Hospital
19th & Hickory Streets 79601</td><td>677-1011</td></tr>
<tr><td>Amarillo</td><td>Poison Control Center
Northwest Texas Hospital
2203 West 6th Street 79106</td><td>376-4431
Ext. 321</td></tr>
<tr><td>Austin</td><td>Poison Control Center, Brackenridge Hospital
14th & Sabine Streets 78701</td><td>478-4490</td></tr>
<tr><td>Beaumont</td><td>Poison Control Center
Baptist Hospital of Southeast Texas
College & 11th Street, Box 1591 77701</td><td>833-7409</td></tr>
<tr><td>Corpus Christi</td><td>Poison Control Center, Memorial Hospital
Medical Library, 2606 Hospital Building
Box 5008 78405</td><td>884-4511
Ext. 273</td></tr>
<tr><td>El Paso</td><td>Poison Control Center
R. E. Thomason General Hospital
4815 Alameda Avenue 79905</td><td>544-1200</td></tr>
<tr><td>Fort Worth</td><td>Poison Control Center
W. I. Cook Memorial Hospital
1212 West Lancaster Avenue 76102</td><td>ED 6-5521
Ext. 17
Night: ED 6-5527</td></tr>
<tr><td>Galveston</td><td>Poison Control Center
Medical Branch Hospital
University of Texas
8th & Mechanic Streets 77550</td><td>765-1420
765-2408</td></tr>
<tr><td>Grand Prairie</td><td>Poison Control Center
Mid-Cities Memorial Hospital
2733 Sherman Road 75050</td><td>264-1651
Ext. 18</td></tr>
<tr><td>Harlingen</td><td>Poison Control Center
Valley Baptist Hospital
2101 South Commerce Street 78550</td><td>423-1224
Ext. 23</td></tr>
<tr><td>Laredo</td><td>Poison Control Center, Mercy Hospital
1515 Logan 78040</td><td>722-2431
Ext. 29</td></tr>
<tr><td>Lubbock</td><td>Poison Control Center, Methodist Hospital
3615 19th Street 79410</td><td>SW 2-1011
Ext. 315</td></tr>
<tr><td>Midland</td><td>Poison Control Center
Midland Memorial Hospital
1908 West Wall 79701</td><td>682-7381
Emergency
Room</td></tr>
<tr><td>Odessa</td><td>Poison Control Center
Medical Center Hospital
600 West 4th Street 79760</td><td>337-7311
Ext. 250</td></tr>
<tr><td>Plainview</td><td>Poison Control Center, Plainview Hospital
2404 Yonkers Street 79072</td><td>296-9601</td></tr>
<tr><td>San Angelo</td><td>Poison Control Center
Shannon West Texas Memorial Hospital
9 South Magdalen Street 76901</td><td>653-6741
Ext. 210</td></tr>
<tr><td>San Antonio</td><td>Poison Control Center
Bexar County Hospital District
7703 Floyd Curl Drive 78229</td><td>223-1481</td></tr>
<tr><td>Texarkana</td><td>Poison Control Center, Wadley Hospital
1000 Pine Street 75501</td><td>793-4511</td></tr>
<tr><td>Tyler</td><td>Poison Control Center
Medical Center Hospital
1000 South Beckham Street 75701</td><td>594-9361
Ext. 255</td></tr>
<tr><td>Waco</td><td>Poison Information Center, Hillcrest Hospital
3000 Herring Avenue 76708</td><td>753-1412</td></tr>
<tr><td>Wharton</td><td>Poison Control Center
Caney Valley Memorial Hospital
503 North Resident Street 77488</td><td>523-2440
Ext. 213
Night: LE 2-1440</td></tr>
<tr><td>Wichita Falls</td><td>Poison Control Center
Wichita General Hospital
Emergency Room, 1600 8th Street 76301</td><td>322-6771</td></tr>
</table>

Utah

<table>
<tr><td></td><td>State Coordinator
State Division of Health
Salt Lake City 84113</td><td>328-6191</td></tr>
<tr><td></td><td>State Division of Health
Salt Lake City 84113</td><td>328-6131</td></tr>
<tr><td>Salt Lake City</td><td>Poison Information Center
University Hospital
University of Utah Medical Center 84112</td><td>328-3711
Ext. 291</td></tr>
</table>

Virgin Islands

State Coordinator
Department of Health, St. Thomas 00801 — 774-1321 Ext. 275

St. Croix
Poison Control Center, Charles Harwood Memorial Hospital, Christiansted 00820 — 773-1212, 773-1311, Ext. 221

Poison Control Center, Ingeborg Nesbitt Clinic, Fredericksted 00840 — 772-0260, 772-0212

St. John
Poison Control Center, Morris F. DeCastro Clinic, Cruz Bay 00830 — 776-1469

St. Thomas
Poison Control Center, Knud-Hansen Memorial Hospital 00801 — 774-1321 Ext. 266

Virginia

State Coordinator
State Department of Health, Richmond 23219 — 644-4111

Alexandria
Poison Control Center, Alexandria Hospital, 709 Duke Street 22314 — 931-2000 Ext. 555

Arlington
Poison Control Center, Arlington Hospital, 5129 North 16th Street 22205 — 524-5900 Ext. 662, 751

Blacksburg
Poison Control Center, Montgomery County Community Hospital, Route 460, South 24060 — 951-1111

Charlottesville
Poison Control Center, University of Virginia Hospital, Box 307, Pediatric Clinic 22903 — 924-2231

Danville
Poison Control Center, Danville Memorial Hospital, 142 South Main Street 22201 — 793-6311 Ext. 257

Falls Church
Poison Control Center, Fairfax Hospital, 3300 Gallows Road 22046 — 698-3111

Hampton
Poison Control Center, Dixie Hospital, Victoria Boulevard 23361 — 722-7921 Ext. 258, 259

Harrisonburg
Poison Control Center, Rockingham Memorial Hospital, 738 South Mason Street 22801 — 434-4421 Ext. 225

Lexington
Poison Control Center, Stonewall Jackson Hospital 22043 — 463-3131

Lynchburg
Poison Control Center, Lynchburg General Marshall Lodge Hospital, Inc., Tate Springs Road 24504 — 846-6511 Ext. 203

Nassawadox
Poison Control Center, Northampton-Accomack Memorial Hospital 23413 — 442-2011

Norfolk
Poison Control Center, Office of Chief Medical Examiner, 427 East Charlotte Street 23510 — 625-1306 Ext. 4, 627-3238

Petersburg
Poison Control Center, Petersburg General Hospital, Mt. Erin & Adams Streets 23803 — 732-7220 Ext. 327, 328

Portsmouth
Poison Control Center, U.S. Naval Hospital 23708 — 397-6581 Ext. 425, 426, 427

Richmond
Poison Information Center, Medical College of Virginia, 1200 East Broad Street 23219 — 770-5123

Roanoke
Poison Control Center, Roanoke Memorial Hospital, Belleview & Lake Avenues 24014 — 342-4541 Ext. 229, 228

Staunton
Poison Control Center, King's Daughters' Hospital, 1410 North Augusta Street 24401 — 885-0361 Ext. 247, 289

Waynesboro
Poison Control Center, Waynesboro Community Hospital, 501 Oak Avenue 22980 — 942-8355 Ext. 436, 440

Williamsburg
Poison Control Center, Williamsburg Community Hospital, Mt. Vernon Avenue, Drawer H 23185 — 229-1120 Ext. 65

Washington

	State Coordinator State Department of Health Olympia 98502	753-5871
Aberdeen	Poison Control Center, St. Joseph's Hospital 1006 North H Street 98520	533-0450 Ext. 42
Olympia	Poison Control Center, St. Peter Hospital 420 South Sherman Street 98502	352-0301
Pasco	Poison Control Center Our Lady of Lourdes Hospital 520 North 4th Avenue 99301	547-7704
Seattle	Poison Control Center Children's Orthopedic Hospital 4800 Sandpoint Way, North East 98105	LA 4-4341
Spokane	Poison Information Center Deaconess Hospital 800 West 5th Avenue 99210	RI 7-4811
Tacoma	Poison Information Center Mary Bridge Children's Hospital 311 South L Street 98405	BR 2-1281 Ext. 59
Vancouver	Poison Control Center St. Joseph Community Hospital 500 East 12th Street 98660	695-4461 Ext. 30

West Virginia

	State Coordinator State Department of Health Charleston 25305	348-2971
Beckley	Poison Control Center, Beckley Hospital 1007 South Oakwood Avenue 25801	252-6431 Ext. 55
Belle	Poison Control Center E. I. DuPont de Nemours & Co. 25015	949-4313 Ext. 261
Charleston	Poison Control Center Charleston General Hospital Elmwood Avenue & Brook Street 25301	348-6286 Ext. 333 Night: 334
	Poison Control Center, Memorial Hospital 3200 Noyes Avenue, South East 25304	348-4211
Clarksburg	Poison Control Center, St. Mary's Hospital Washington & Chestnut Streets 26301	623-3444 Ext. 251
Huntington	Poison Control Center Cabell-Huntington Hospital 1340 16th Street 25701	696-6160 696-6161
	Poison Control Center, St. Mary's Hospital 2900 1st Avenue 25701	696-3762
Martinsburg	Poison Control Center King's Daughters' Hospital 25401	267-8981 Ext. 201
Morgantown	Poison Control Center West Virginia University Hospital 26506	293-4451 Night: 293-5341
Parkersburg	Poison Control Center Camden-Clark Hospital 717 Ann Street 26101	428-8011 Ext. 28 131
	Poison Control Center, St. Joseph's Hospital 19th Street & Murdoch Avenue 26101	422-8535 Ext. 251
Ronceverte	Poison Control Center Greenbrier Valley Hospital 608 Greenbrier Avenue 24970	647-4411 647-4412 647-4413
Weirton	Poison Control Center Weirton General Hospital St. John Road 26062	748-3232 Ext. 208
Weston	Poison Control Center Stonewall Jackson Hospital 504 Main 26452	269-3000
Wheeling	Poison Control Center, Wheeling Hospital 109 Main Street 26003	233-4455 Ext. 224, 203

Wisconsin

	State Coordinator Department of Health and Social Services Madison 53701	266-1511
Eau Claire	Poison Control Center, Luther Hospital 310 Chestnut Street 54701	832-6611 Ext. 227

Green Bay	Poison Information Center Bellin Memorial Hospital 744 South Webster Avenue 54301	437-9031 Ext. 257
Kenosha	Poison Control Center, Kenosha Hospital 6308 8th Avenue 53140	656-2201
Madison	Poison Information Center University Hospital Dept. of Pharmacology 1300 University Avenue 53706	262-3702
Milwaukee	Poison Control Center Milwaukee Children's Hospital 1700 West Wisconsin 53233	344-7100 Ext. 308

Wyoming

	State Coordinator State Department of Public Health Cheyenne 82001	777-7275
Casper	Poison Control Center Natrona County Hospital 1233 East 2nd Street 82601	235-1311 Ext. 131
Cheyenne	Poison Control Center Laramie County Memorial Hospital 23rd & House Streets 82001	634-3341 Ext. 238

Notes